I Can Still Laugh

STORIES OF INSPIRATION AND HOPE FROM
INDIVIDUALS LIVING WITH ALZHEIMER'S

Audette Rackley

Audette Rackley

with

Sophia Dembling

Center for BrainHealth
The University of Texas at Dallas
2200 West Mockingbird Lane
Dallas, Texas 75235
www.centerforbrainhealth.com
214-905-3007

ISBN: 1-4392-3939-8
ISBN-13: 9781439239391

PRINTED IN THE UNITED STATES OF AMERICA

Acknowledgements

This book would not be possible without generous support from:

Friends of Temple and Anne Stark

Bert Headden

Friends of Retired Admiral Wayne and Molly Smith

Our deepest gratitude goes to the Stark Club, their wives, and children for sharing their stories in the hope of helping others. This book is in your hands because they had a strong desire to "make a difference for the people who would come after them."

The Stark Club dedicates this book to everyone who might find inspiration and hope in their stories.

Contents

Introduction

Chapter 1 **The Stark Reality of Alzheimer's** **21**
Everyone who met Temple Stark was his friend, before and after he was diagnosed with Alzheimer's disease.

Chapter 2 **Genius of Blessing** **37**
When Jerry Roach's life looked most bleak and hopeless, an angel appeared and adopted him.

Chapter 3 **Facing Down Fear with Fun** **49**
Alzheimer's disease didn't rob Jay Haberman of the twinkle in his eyes or his jolly approach to life.

Chapter 4 **Meaning Beyond Words** **59**
Creativity is the engine that still drives Jodi Madigan's life despite Primary Progressive Aphasia.

Chapter 5 **From Anger to Activism** **71**
First Bill Crist was angry about his Lewy body syndrome, then he channeled that energy into helping others.

Chapter 6   **Detoxifying the Fear of Dementia   81**
Semantic dementia is difficult to diagnose, but once Bob Eshbaugh knew what he faced, he did so with grace and charm.

Chapter 7   **Wholeness from Despair   93**
When Bill Tuel finally admitted the troubles Alzheimer's was causing him, he reclaimed his place as pillar of his family.

Chapter 8   **Engineering Hope   107**
With his methodical, problem-solving mind, Jack Kalling invents ways to work around Primary Progressive Aphasia.

Chapter 9   **Seize the Day   119**
Stan Fedyniak found time for pleasant new pursuits when Lewy body disease forced him to slow his pace.

Chapter 10   **Staying the Course   129**
Quiet, athletic Tom Keppler didn't forsake the physical activities he loved after a diagnosis of Alzheimer's disease.

Chapter 11   **A Journey of Love   141**
Love of family defined Delbert Duncan and family made sure he was never alone with his Alzheimer's disease.

Chapter 12   **A Natural Leader   151**
The qualities that made Wayne Smith the kind of man people loved and respected were not dimmed by Primary Progressive Aphasia.

Chapter 13 **A Generous Life** **161**
Frances Goad Cecil lived her life with an
open heart and irrepressible verve and
Alzheimer's disease couldn't change that.

Chapter 14 **Reframing Dementia** **171**
Stark Club members prove that life does
not end with a diagnosis. They hope you
will find hope and strength in their stories.

Introduction

Every two weeks, a group of people dealing with various forms of progressive dementia come together for ninety minutes, bringing with them courage, optimism, and strength.

Most members of the Stark Club, named for its dynamic founding member, Temple Stark, have Alzheimer's disease. Others have such diseases as Primary Progressive Aphasia, which affects grammar and semantics, or Semantic dementia, which affects one's memory of objects and their labels.

When many of us think of dementia, we imagine elderly people. But all of the members of the Stark Club are in their fifties and sixties and have young-age-onset dementia (except one special older member whom you will read about later). The diseases hit at a time in their lives when they were still vital and active. All were still employed and in their peak earning years when they started showing symptoms. They were waiting for children to graduate high school or college, looking forward to weddings and grandkids, and certainly not ready to retire. Young, energetic, and passionate, they maintained a desire to make meaningful contributions to life.

In these pages, you will meet some of the inspirational members of the Stark Club and the caregivers and family members supporting them throughout their disease progression. These individuals have many lessons to share, including practical wisdom and tactical strategies that have helped them to stay engaged, maintain dignity, preserve hope, and focus on what a person with dementia *can* do with the rest of his or her life.

––––––

I came to know the astonishing members of the Stark Club through my job at The University of Texas at Dallas Center for BrainHealth. I have a master's degree in communication disorders and became interested in dementia after taking an elective course taught by the center's executive director, Dr. Sandra Chapman. I was fortunate to lead a research project evaluating the effects of cognitive stimulation on individuals with Alzheimer's disease. The study showed positive benefits, but the most impressive benefits really became clear to me through my work with the Stark Club.

The diagnosis of any form of dementia is terrifying. While research into causes and treatment of dementia is at the forefront for the brain science community, these diseases are still only barely treatable and they remain incurable. But when most people think of these diseases, they also think only of the end stages. At the Center for BrainHealth, we help people see the wealth of possibilities for fulfilling lives in the midst of the disease. Our focus is to help individuals and families continue an active and engaged life for as long as possible. Even more important, our research has found that staying active, connected, and cognitively stimulated in the early stages may help slow the progression of the symptoms.

Temple Stark is a great example of this. For years after he received his diagnosis, "we did an awful lot of stuff and kept our lives happy and wonderful," says his wife, Anne, whose abundant warmth and energy match that of her husband. "It's not a death sentence. Your lives can be really rich and fulfilled and happy and you can savor what you have during those months and years." While, of course, life changed after the diagnosis, "we don't act like there's something wrong. I think that's what kept him going as long as he's been going."

Members of the Stark Club strongly believe the disease is not the main culprit that robs them of who they are. Much worse is the way people pull away because they are uncomfortable and unsure how to behave around the person with dementia. Involvement in the Stark Club helps keep members and their loved ones involved and life-affirming.

It was a Stark Club member, Bill Tuel, who suggested that the group leave a legacy by publishing this book. "We have some pretty interesting and inspiring stories. We should write our own book," Bill said one day, as the Stark Club discussed Tom Brokaw's book *The Greatest Generation*, which contains the stories of World War II veterans. And from that almost offhand comment, this book was born. With it, members of the Stark Club hope to help other people diagnosed with dementia bring more to their own lives. They have taken this on as a mission.

———

Stark Club members are men and women accustomed to being in control and in charge. They are well traveled, well read professionals who are far from ready to settle down.

The Stark Club is not a support group; it is an intervention program based on research and an understanding of the effects of the disease on the brain and how to optimize functioning. This is no pity party and there's nothing touchy-feely about it—unless you count the genuine warmth and affection that flows among its members.

While the official meetings take place at the Center for BrainHealth, the connections between its members have long since sprung the bounds of the building. Stark Club members and their families socialize often, including parties, standing lunch dates, and other get-togethers. These men and women have found a safe place and stimulating company with each other.

"The Stark Club gives back a piece of self confidence Delbert lost in the final months he was on the job," says Judy Duncan, wife of Delbert Duncan, a retired supermarket executive diagnosed with Alzheimer's.

The Stark Club is a discussion-based program and my role is to engage these intelligent men and women. I must admit, I often learn more from them than they do from me. People with Alzheimer's disease still have a lot to say—their passions, interests, desires, and world knowledge are still a part of them. These are some of the most intelligent people I know. Their memories may be affected, but they still want to talk about interesting topics—politics, history, research.

The Stark Club represents a new way of treating people with progressive dementia, with its unique emphasis on the early stages, that may help slow the progression of the symptoms.

The research I helped conduct with Dr. Chapman examined the effects of "cognitive-communication stimulation" on individuals with Alzheimer's who were also being treated with the common drug, Aricept (the research was funded by Pfizer and Eisai, which makes the drug). We studied fifty-four individuals with mild Alzheimer's disease, treating a random sample of half with medication only and the other half with medication plus cognitive-communication stimulation, similar to the discussions we have in the Stark Club.

While admittedly neither drugs nor stimulation cure or halt the progress of the disease, our results clearly indicated—and in a relatively short time—that the combination of medication and stimulation may slow the declines in patients' discourse (conversational) abilities, functional abilities, emotional symptoms, and overall global performance. *In other words, people who received both the medication and cognitive stimulation experienced lesser declines in their abilities and emotional well being than people who received the medication only.*

If you are currently dealing with a recent diagnosis, this is important information because it tells you that you have some control over your situation. While you will have hard times—and coming to terms with the diagnosis is certainly one of them—focusing on what you or a loved one with dementia *can* do instead of what he or she *can't* do makes the best of the hand you've been dealt, and may help slow the progression of symptoms.

We look at it this way: If someone has a stroke and can't move his right arm, we help him use his left arm. The same goes for Alzheimer's—if a person can't remember new details, for example, we help him use his wisdom.

———

When a dementia diagnosis is made, the patient is typically prescribed medication and told, "There's really nothing else we can do. See you in six months to a year."

This dismissal is devastating. Patients and their families feel powerless, as if all they can do is sit at home and wait for the worst. At the Center for BrainHealth, we saw a big gap in treatment options at the early stage, when most people desperately need information and hope. The Stark Club's cognitive-communication stimulation approach helps to bridge this gap.

After diagnosis, one of the first problems many individuals face is fear—fear of saying something foolish in public, fear of repeating themselves or something others have said, fear of losing track of conversations. Many people with dementia have told me that if a conversation would just slow down they could keep up, but the pace of the average conversation is many times too fast for them to process. As a result, even though they are still capable of staying engaged, people in early stages often begin to withdraw.

In the Stark Club, we modify the environment, slowing the pace of discussion to allow for processing time. We develop topics instead of jumping from topic to topic, and invite people into the discussion instead of leaving them to fend for themselves. We seek out topics that will be of interest to group members and will help trigger memories. And when we discuss information related to Alzheimer's, we break it all down carefully to provide base information they can build on.

Because of these considerations, Stark Club members find they can enjoy participation instead of being fearful. And when value is placed on each person's individual contribution, and the group topics are chosen in such a way to tap world knowledge and highlight individual interests, you'd be amazed at the direction and depth of the conversation. One visitor to the group remarked, "If you had not told me, I would think this is a group of board members."

One valuable component of the intervention programs is the creation of a *Collection of Life Stories* book for each participant. While the concept of creating memory books for individuals with dementia is not new, often these books are limited to just the facts—date and place of birth, family names, job histories, etc.—and typically are not created until individuals with dementia are unable to tell stories on their own. However, for our version of the memory books, we engage individuals in the early stages of the disease to tell their own stories. We draw from their long-term memories to tell the really important stories of their lives—their proudest moments, fondest memories, funny situations they recall, and the people, activities, and events of their lives that made them who they are. Each story, told in the person's own words, is paired with an appropriate picture in a binder. These books help keep people grounded with who they are beyond the disease. The books help keep doors of communication open between individuals with Alzheimer's and the people around them, providing them with a way to interact. Often, even in late stages of dementia, hearing the stories from their books triggers recognition and can be a stimulus for continued interaction at holidays or during family visits.

We also help members focus on using the abilities they retain through a variety of activities, including continuing to pursue hobbies and encouraging volunteerism—for instance, reading to children in a Head Start program, building wheelchair ramps for people's homes, delivering

Meals on Wheels, serving as a nursing home ombudsmen, stocking food pantries, or serving as a greeter at a senior center. Focusing on what each Stark Club member *can* do and enjoy contributes immeasurably to each individual's sense of purpose and quality of life.

————

If you are reading this book, you are probably either coping with dementia or working with dementia patients. If you are a family member, you might be frightened, unsure, fearful, and angry that the person you know and love has been snatched from you.

Living with dementia is hard. The purpose of this book is to provide a fresh perspective. The challenges are real, but instead of focusing on those, we want to provide people with tools to build positive things in their lives in the midst of dementia. We seek to reframe the disease to help people see the possibilities for positive experiences.

I hope you will find comfort in meeting the members of the Stark Club and their caregivers, who can show you how much life remains after a diagnosis of progressive dementia. Yes, you are at the beginning of a long and often difficult road, but so too is dealing with cancer, congestive heart problems, or lung disease.

In the stories in this book, you will see that there is still joy to be found even amidst the sadness and stress. And you will see that despite the changes that occur over the course of dementia, there is an essence in each individual that remains constant. Even as his disease progresses, Temple Stark gets no greater joy than from being in a social situation, surrounded by people and laughing the big, happy laugh that people love him for. That has always been his core personality and it never changed.

"I wish people would not look at me with so much sadness and pity when I tell them I have Alzheimer's," Temple told *The Dallas Morning News* in 2003. "Some immediately have tears. That is one of the hardest things to deal with. I just wish they knew that I am not losing my mind and that I can still laugh."

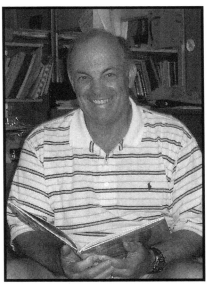

Temple Stark

Everyone who met Temple Stark was his friend, before and after he was diagnosed with Alzheimer's disease.

Chapter 1
The Stark Reality of
Alzheimer's

*"There's nothing worse than being lonely.
It's not good for you." Temple Stark*

Temple Stark is all about charisma and always has been. He was a state champion football player in high school, big man on campus—including serving as president of his fraternity—at The University of Texas, an Air Force pilot, and a successful insurance underwriter. Despite Alzheimer's disease, Temple remains the kind of guy who never met a stranger.

Temple and his wife Anne both secretly and silently suspected the worst, but decided to just keep to business as usual until they knew for sure. Anne went with Temple for his neurological evaluation, but she returned to the doctor alone for the diagnosis because Temple was away. The doctor was blunt. He told Anne that Temple had Alzheimer's disease and would die in a nursing home.

Despite her previous suspicions, this blunt delivery of the news stunned and terrified Anne.

Anne absorbed the news as best she could before telling Temple.

"First. I went to a close friend's house. I slugged back about three glasses of wine and we talked and cried and talked and cried," Anne says. "Then I called my parents and cried some more."

Then Anne and their sixteen-year-old daughter, Mary Ellen, drove three hours to the lakeside cabin where Temple was staying on a guys' getaway. (Daughter Katie, then nineteen, was in Florida and Anne didn't want to deliver news this devastating over the telephone, she waited until Katie was home to tell her.)

"When I got to the lake, I hugged and kissed Temple and said, 'I've got your diagnosis.'" Anne says. Then she broke the news to him.

Anne and Mary Ellen stayed at the lake that night. "At five o'clock the next morning, I turned over and looked at him," Anne says. "His eyes were wide open. I said, 'What are you doing awake?' He said, 'I didn't think I ought to be sleeping.'"

Anne and Temple told the other men in the group, and decided Temple should finish out the guys-only weekend. He returned home Sunday and began making plans for his retirement. Temple was fifty-four years old.

———

The thing I've noticed most sitting at the table with Temple during meetings of the Stark Club is his strong social abilities. Whether he is able to clearly communicate his thoughts or not, his warm and engaging spirit comes through loud and clear. Temple is the kind of guy who makes everyone feel special. Everyone feels he's their best friend.

Temple's gift for making friends everywhere he goes is legendary. So the Starks' life was full and very busy when Temple first started showing symptoms of Alzheimer's. Temple was a successful underwriter, an avid golfer, and active in the Salesmanship Club, a service organization in Dallas dedicated to helping young people. Anne had a law practice.

"Our lives were so fast-paced at that point," Anne recalls. "Katie was a senior, and Mary Ellen was a freshman in high school. Temple was busy. I was in litigation. We had a really good social life—lots of people, lots of friends. We traveled a lot."

It was friends who noticed Temple's lapses first: Temple increasingly forgetting things. Struggling at bridge. Losing his focus at work. One after another, friends pulled Anne aside and asked if she had noticed, urged her to have him tested, pushed against what Anne now admits was her denial.

"Funny—when you have a really, really close marriage, as we always did … I never had talked about Temple behind his back," Anne says. "I never even thought of him as a separate human being from me.

"How was I going to say this to him? How am I going to tell him to get tested without it threatening his entire being? Finally, one morning, as he was waking up, I sat down on the bed and told him what friends had said: There's something wrong and you need to get tested. He got very defensive, and I started crying. And when I start crying, he'll do whatever I want him to do."

"Once you make a step like that, you need to act right away," Anne says—and they did, seeing a neurologist within days. "That was the first time I had any sort of a grip on Temple's deficits at that time," Anne says. "The doctor asked Temple to draw a face on a clock at 3:30 and he couldn't do it. I'm sitting there, watching, and I'm just stunned. Temple was the first guy in our neighborhood and among all our friends to have a computer at home. He did spreadsheets and he taught himself everything."

———

A friend told Anne and Temple about Sandi (Dr. Chapman) and the Center for BrainHealth. At that time, we had seen a number of younger men coming through with Alzheimer's and other forms of dementia, but could find little existing information and intervention techniques available to help them. I had already started working with younger men. Temple was one of the youngest men we had ever worked with at that time.

Within a year, Temple stopped driving, although he retained other abilities for a long time—reading, for example, and his ability to relate to people. From the very beginning, the Starks were proactive, making sure Temple stayed busy and engaged. Jennifer Zientz, one of our clinicians who was part of Temple's diagnostic team, remembers Anne calling frequently, asking about things Temple could and couldn't do. "Seeing what they were dealing with—that here was somebody at the top of his earning potential, having to stop working, facing this disease—we felt warranted a whole new set of rules," Jennifer says.

And so the center tried brought together four younger men with dementia, and the Young Men's Club—the first version of the Stark Club—took shape in 2001.

For Temple, joining a group of other men was natural—he was a joiner and loved hanging out with male friends. The other members of the group called Temple "the professor" because his knowledge was so wide-ranging, and he was always the first to bring in articles about new research. "If you didn't stay three steps ahead of him, he was ten steps ahead of you in what he read," Sandi recalls.

At the same time, because reading remained among Temple's strengths, Jennifer and a doctoral student who was working with her arranged for him to read to children with hearing problems at the Callier Center for Communication Disorders, which is also part of The University of Texas at Dallas. Temple, with typical good humor, said it was a perfect setup because, "I can't read and they can't hear!" The children adored Temple, and the feeling was mutual. When he walked in the door, all the kids ran up to him. And when one of the kids corrected him while he was reading, Temple began encouraging the kids to read to him, taking his challenges in stride and good-naturedly accepting help even from children, without feeling compelled to prove anything to anyone.

This weekly rendezvous with the kids, which he sometimes referred to as his job, was important to Temple. As Anne observed, people like Temple in the early stages of Alzheimer's disease are a huge, untapped volunteer resource. Young, energetic, vital, still in possession of many useful skills, they are able, willing, and anxious to contribute and provide services in any way they can—and they can do a lot, as Temple and other members of the Stark Club prove again and again.

Around this time, Sandi and Temple made a presentation about Alzheimer's to the Salesmanship Club. "Seventy-five percent of the people didn't know he had

Alzheimer's disease," Sandi recalls. "When I said he had it, the whole room gasped. Then Temple got up and gave a very moving speech. He said, 'People look at me and they feel sorry for me, but don't. I'm getting to do everything now I can possibly dream of. Which one of you gets to play golf every day?'

"Temple told the group about his first symptoms, about how he was having trouble understanding documents at work, and he pointed out that he had always been good with people and still was. He said that people's reactions to the diagnosis are worse than the disease itself because he most wanted everyone to continue seeing him as a person, not just an Alzheimer's patient. And he ended with a joke. He said, 'We've been playing golf for a long time. I hope that each of you will still help me play golf until the last day. You may have to turn me in the right direction, you might have to keep score, but I'll still beat you.'"

Moved almost to tears by Temple's forthrightness, his calm and reassuring acceptance of his diagnosis, and his ability to joke even in the face of it, Temple's audience leapt to its feet, giving him the first standing ovation that the club had ever given a speaker. Temple had set the tone for how these people would continue viewing him and Alzheimer's disease. They would never think of the disease in the same way again.

Temple's openness about the disease has been enormously helpful to his friends as they come to terms with the diagnosis. In my experience, people who deal openly with the disease and are willing to ask for help and acknowledge their challenges tend to function better. The stress created by trying to keep a diagnosis a secret adds tremendous pressure and—like any stress for people with Alzheimer's—can actually further impair functioning.

Temple's friend Sherri Pulliam remembers driving with Temple to the Starks' lakehouse not long after his diagnosis. "We had been friends for so long, that I couldn't pretend that I didn't know about the diagnosis," she says. "I just came right out and asked him how he felt about it. He was so open and honest and we talked about it. He said he felt badly for Anne and his two daughters because they would be carrying the 'load.' He said he didn't feel badly for himself because he would eventually not know what was happening to him. I asked him about the tests that he had to take for the diagnosis and he told me about each one—always making me laugh, even then, with his great sense of humor. After about twenty minutes on the topic, he changed the subject and we both began to reminisce about all of our adventures and misadventures in college. It was the best three hours I have spent with Temple in many years, because I had him all to myself with no distractions and no one else telling stories but him and me. We laughed and remembered for hours."

By being open and straightforward with Sherri about his diagnosis, fears, and challenges, Temple put her at ease and they were able move past it quickly into more pleasant topics.

Even children are able to understand and cope well with more than we imagine. Frieda Clark, a friend of the Starks, tells a wonderful story about her five-year-old son Andrew. "Anne and I discussed for a long time what to say to my son about Temple's disease," Frieda recalls. "I first told him about Alzheimer's, but at that time Temple was still a long way from where he is today. Andrew said little. Then, while we were watching television one night, a special came on about Alzheimer's. I was about to change the channel, but Andrew said no, he wanted to watch it. It was a terrific way for him to learn from a medical standpoint about Temple and Alzheimer's. From that day forward, Andrew has been amazing and looks so forward to the time he spends with Temple."

———

Temple continued reading to the children at the Callier Center and we adjusted the reading level of the books as his reading skills diminished. After about two years, however, we could see him becoming hesitant and backing off when the books were too difficult. He was frustrated both by his reading struggles and because of the distraction of all the children climbing on him. His attention was getting worse and he was getting agitated. When the reading finally was clearly too much for him to enjoy any more, we ended that and focused more on his interactions in the Stark Club.

All along, Anne was an ideal helpmate to Temple. The couple was fortunate in that Temple's disability insurance was about equal to his salary, and this allowed Anne to continue working and hire a part-time companion/caregiver for Temple, which took a great deal of stress off her. The family also took several trips together after the diagnosis, including one to Italy. An ID bracelet for peace of mind, and cooperation among Anne and their daughters keeping track of Temple, allowed the trip to go on without a hitch—except the time Temple got left behind at a train station as the train doors closed in preparation to pull out. Fortunately, Anne got the conductor's attention in time to get Temple safely back on board. (Even though, in her panic, she called the male conductor "Senora.")

Throughout the early- and mid-stages of the disease, many friends Temple made over the years have helped make sure this sociable man stays busy and never gets lonely. Every Thursday, friends from the Salesmanship Club pick Temple up to take him to the club luncheon meetings. Because people with Alzheimer's thrive on routine, weekends away with the guys became too stressful for Temple about two years after his diagnosis, but four years after his diagnosis he continues to join his buddies on golfing day trips. Although he can't golf as he used to do, Temple continues to enjoy the camaraderie. "He wakes up smiling and whistling on those days," Anne says. These trips allow Temple to enjoy a sense of normalcy even if his level of participation has changed.

Anne admits that their social life was curtailed some—and increasingly as the disease takes a greater toll on Temple's functioning—but they retain a core group of friends, and socializing remains among Temple's greatest joys. "His memory for the people in his life is great," Anne says. "There's nobody that I've talked to him about that he hasn't been able to identify. He forgets names, but he knows who they are."

This social interaction is clearly important and beneficial to Temple. "I truly believe that one of the reasons Temple has done so well is that Anne takes him everywhere, has guests and parties at their home often, and makes sure he keeps up with his friends," Sherri Pulliam says.

And to his friends' great credit, they have stared down the discomfort that so many people feel when dealing with individuals with Alzheimer's to find that the man they loved remains as loveable as ever. Most important, they meet Temple on ground that's comfortable for him. Four years after his diagnosis, Temple is no longer able to carry on in-depth conversations and so his friends have stopped trying to engage him in high-level discussions, but they do not shy from engaging him at all. Instead, they find Temple's comfort zone and settle in there with him. Sometimes it means just being goofy. Sometimes it's reminding Temple of his own stories, which he quite often recognizes and enjoys hearing again.

In the Stark Club, we spent a number of meetings talking about each of the members in turn. When it was Temple's turn, we used his *Collection of Life Stories* book (described in the Introduction) and stories Anne and his friends told us to assist Temple in recounting some of his wild and hilarious tales. The group laughed until they cried. Temple with a huge grin on his face, kept asking "How do you know all this stuff?" but clearly understood that the stories were his.

And here is another aspect of Temple's personality that has remained strong, even if he requires support. "Temple is probably one of the best storytellers I have ever been around," says Temple's friend Bruce Sifford. "He has countless tales of jet fighters, whisky drinking and more. I could listen to him all day, any day."

Temple's ability to remember his stories is impaired, but with proper support, he can continue regaling people with his tales through what we call story partnering, where someone who knows the stories provides prompts and guidance that creates a framework for the person with Alzheimer's to fill in as much of his or her own stories as possible. In the Stark Club, students study up on individual members before we meet so they can partner with the member in their storytelling.

Temple's friend Gregg Lafitte explains that the silly friendship he has always had with Temple is still fun. "Temple and I developed a relationship that included lots of messing with each other," he says. "We would gig each other, make stupid faces, talk stupid—a lot of which stemmed from his role in our rookie Salesmanship Club skit, when he played Forrest Gump. The interesting thing to me is no matter what has left Temple, those funny antics remain. We'll go to lunch now and spend the entire time laughing our butts off. The subject matter makes no sense and a third party observer would think we had both lost our marbles, but the important thing is what remains: his humor and appreciation for life and what he gives me— himself, open and honest."

Temple's friend Coley Clark says, "We talk about things that happened thirty years ago. He can't exactly respond coherently—though once in a while he throws out a zinger that is right on the mark—but he definitely relates. We laugh a lot, and any joke I tell he thinks is funny. Last time we went out, I put on an oldies station and he can sing every word, which I also found amazing. So we sing together as loud as we can."

Even five-year-old Andrew Clark understands the concept of accepting Temple for what he can do rather than what he can't. "What has truly amazed me is how he accepts Temple for the man he is and relishes his minor accomplishments," says Andrew's mother, Frieda. "Whenever Temple remembers something or whistles a tune, my son will wink at me and then later say, 'Mom, that is really good that Temple could remember that.'"

This story is important to me because sometimes what is obvious to children may not be as obvious to adults. Too often, we focus on what the individual is losing instead of acknowledging and appreciating abilities retained. At the center, we try to help caregivers focus on the retained abilities. Until there is a cure or a treatment to stop the progression of the disease, decline is inevitable. In a year, caregivers and people with Alzheimer's may look back wistfully on the abilities retained today. Keeping focused on retained strengths and making small changes along the way helps everyone to cope with the march of the disease and is much preferable to over-adjusting too quickly by limiting interactions with the world, or denying the need for change and later having to make huge adjustments all at once.

The sensitivity friends show to Temple and their expanded understanding of communication is exactly what we wish for the individuals we work with. Anne advises people before they spend time with him that they will have to look after Temple and adjust their expectations of him. "I've talked a little bit about comprehension being low, and don't expect long conversations," she says. "Otherwise, he's not difficult to be around. If he's with other people, he's normally very happy." And if Temple seems agitated or stressed out, there is often a very good reason, such as a time when a friend escorted him to the men's room, but didn't realize he needed more help than that.

"I now have to get his food for him when we go through the buffet line at the Salesmanship Club lunch and lead him to the table, but once I put the right utensils in his hand, he can eat," Clark says. "If I tell him to wipe his face or not put his fork on my plate, he takes it well and just laughs. Sometimes I tell stories about Temple that he has told me ... things that happened to him in college and he will maybe, maybe add something, or try to, but he laughs regardless. He's still a great guy, and though you have to watch him carefully, fun to be with."

———

Of course, not everything is beautiful in the way it once was. Though Anne's love for Temple is still deeply felt, their relationship, of necessity, changed. Four years after Temple's diagnosis, Anne says her marriage is a mere shadow of what it was.

"I hate to say this, but we don't have a marriage in any sense—physical or emotional—any more," Anne says with sorrow but no self-pity. "I love Temple and will always love him and will always take care of him, but at this point I am more like a parent. You can't prepare yourself for this. My self-protection mechanism is to focus on the joy in other things—my children, my job, my friends. If he's well taken care of and if he's happy, I'm OK. That's been my response all along. It's not about me. It's about him. If he's OK, I'm OK. I can handle it if he's happy. I just put my emotions over here, on hold. And I know we have so much more than a lot of people."

Anne and Temple's daughters also have had an enormous and difficult adjustment to make. "I tried to shield them in the beginning," Anne says. "But I think it's matured both of them. And I've learned how very compassionate they both are. There is a closeness that comes with this type of struggle that many families may never feel. Katie and Mary Ellen have matured beyond their years in ways I wish we could have spared them, but that experience will serve them well in years to come."

At twenty years old, Mary Ellen does display mature wisdom about the difficult path she has been forced to walk. "From the first day we found out about Dad's diagnosis, an onlooker probably would have thought it was any one of us but dad who had Alzheimer's," she says. "He probably thought it over a second and then went on his way. My mom, sister, and I didn't take the news so lightly. I thought mostly about losing my dad before I had ever really gotten to know him. What I didn't know was that I was about to learn so much from him. His reaction to the diagnosis was just the beginning. From that day on, I have seen a man take a life-altering disease and just knock it right down. I have seen a man take every one of his days and live it to the fullest. And I have never seen a man so content, so happy—always smiling, laughing, or playing around."

"My dad has faced his illness head-on and with an attitude of hope, love, and bravery," Katie says. "I hope that I have learned from him and can live my life with some of the genuine goodness he possesses."

And so this close-knit family continues braving the disease with courage, love, and optimism.

"One of the fascinating aspects of this journey is our adaptability," Anne says. "No matter how difficult the losses become, each day brings some hope and some joy,"

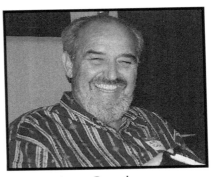

Jerry Roach

When Jerry Roach's life looked most bleak and hopeless, an angel appeared and adopted him.

Chapter 2
Genius of Blessing

"Alzheimer's isn't that bad.
I can have vanilla ice cream for the first time
every day!" Jerry Roach

Jerry Roach is smart. A whiz at math, Jerry was an architectural and structural engineer who designed buildings all over the country, including a robotics plant at Sandia National Laboratories and the Sea Island Hilton. Yet the first thing people notice about Jerry is not his intellect, but his warmth. He greets everyone with a handshake or hug, and he always has a joke to tell, followed by his contagious laugh. Jerry's joy and optimism are indomitable.

Knowing how to get from point A to point B can sometimes be daunting. The journey with Alzheimer's is different for everyone and the path is never a straight line. There are moments when people feel overwhelmed, even paralyzed by looming issues.

Enter Jerry Roach, optimist. Even after his diagnosis, Jerry has an incredible ability to focus on his objective instead of his perceived limitations. His warm nature reaches out to people and inspires them to reach back. One person told me, "He could make friends with a fencepost." And even as life threw challenge after challenge in his path, Jerry never lost his spirit. His perspective is one to learn from. He finds hope in the midst of challenges and always believes something good is ahead. He does not wait for life to come to him—he pursues it.

Joan Eades didn't have to go on a date with Jerry—who was a widower—after they met in church. She didn't have to make him her friend after he told her he had Alzheimer's disease. She didn't have to volunteer to help Jerry's twenty-three-year-old daughter, Stephanie, with his care, and she certainly didn't have to move Jerry into her home with her, allowing Stephanie to move to Chicago and get on with her young life knowing her father was in capable and caring hands.

But Joan did all that, both because her strong faith told her to and because Jerry's loving and generous soul reached out to touch hers. Jerry was unafraid of presenting himself openly and honestly to Joan, and she recognized immediately that he was a kind, good, and loving man who needed the strength she was able to offer.

But let's start at the beginning.

———

I met Jerry and his wife, Charlotte, after his diagnosis at the age of fifty-four. He was in my very first Alzheimer's intervention group. Tragically, in January 2001, eighteen months after Jerry came to the Center for BrainHealth, Charlotte contracted autoimmune hepatitis, and within three weeks had passed away.

Jerry met Charlotte at Baylor University in Waco, Texas. In a bold and typically optimistic move, Jerry had decided to work his way through Charlotte's dorm, asking every woman in it to go out with him.

"He wasn't to my mom's room yet, and so she asked him out," Stephanie says. "It was fairly common knowledge that he was dating everyone in the dorm."

The two became a couple sometime during Jerry's sophomore year. They married after graduation, and Jerry launched his career as an architectural and structural engineer; he loved to drive around Dallas and point out buildings he helped build. Even after his diagnosis, this was a proud pastime for him.

For a while in the late 1980s, Jerry had his own engineering firm, although Stephanie recalls this time as a mixed blessing because he was working so hard. "I clearly remember sleeping under the drafting tables. He was great at the drafting part, the architectural engineer part. But bookkeeping and paying people and making sure he kept the lights on were hard. He had employees—four or five at one time—and had regular employee problems, but he was too nice a guy to fire people and be tough. He never wanted to hurt anyone's feelings."

And that wasn't the only challenge in the family's life at that time. The reason Stephanie was at her dad's office so much was because Charlotte had suffered a nervous breakdown and was hospitalized from the time Stephanie was in third grade until she was in fifth grade.

Jerry ultimately shut down his business and got another job, but it was at that time the job problems started. First, Jerry was affected by downsizing. But then other problems started affecting his career. Since Stephanie was young and then left home for college, she didn't know exactly what was going wrong, but she remembers rough patches. She remembers not being surprised when she heard her dad had lost another job. She knew that his job reviews were not as good as they once had been. As technology changed his field, Jerry was unable to master computers in order to keep up. "He went from being able to design a building to not being able to inspect a building," Stephanie says. "He couldn't even make sure that he completed all he needed to do. That made it kind of obvious that there was something wrong."

Charlotte kept Stephanie apprised of some of the problems, but she also protected her daughter. "I wasn't aware of how important it all was at the time," Stephanie recalls—although she knew things were going wrong somehow. "He would get frustrated and borderline violent whenever he had no idea what was going on." Nobody realized it at the time, but Jerry's mounting frustration was due to more than a string of lost jobs and financial difficulties. The subtle symptoms of Alzheimer's disease were mounting.

In the course of their struggles, Jerry and Charlotte lost their home and, ultimately, had to file bankruptcy. All the while, Jerry was seeing doctors and undergoing tests, trying to figure out why he was failing at tasks that previously had been no problem. The month Stephanie was to graduate from Baylor and move back in with her parents, doctors at the UT Southwestern Medical Center diagnosed Jerry with Alzheimer's disease.

And, as we see happen so many times, that helped ease some of the intense stress Jerry was feeling about what previously had been the "problem with no name." Suddenly, all the anger and abusiveness dissipated. "After he knew what was going on, that all went away," Stephanie says. "You could tell the difference in one day to the next."

And the Jerry everyone loved best was back.

Still, financial conditions for the family remained difficult. They were crammed into a small apartment and living close to the bone, finding opportunities to earn money wherever they could—for example, by participating in paid clinical studies.

That is how Jerry and Charlotte came to the Center for BrainHealth in 1999 as part of a research study evaluating the combined effects of cognitive stimulation and drug intervention. And so Jerry became part of what would ultimately develop into the Stark Club, and he helped set the tone of warmth and acceptance that is the group's hallmark.

In this early research study group, Jerry immediately established friendships with other group members. Even though the other members were more impaired than he, Jerry always saw the person, not the impairment. He was always ready to make a friend and to reach out and help with a smile on his face. He was and is one of the warmest human beings you could ever hope to meet—an amazingly gracious and friendly man.

Jerry and Charlotte became excellent spokespeople for Alzheimer's; they even appeared in television news programs talking about the disease. Jerry was never shy about telling people he had Alzheimer's, which makes a powerful statement to a world that can sometimes treat the disease as something to hide.

And Jerry didn't hide himself away after his diagnosis. In the early stages of the disease, he got a job at a local senior center within walking distance from his home. He helped serve lunch, and this routine not only kept him active and connected, but was a way to give back to the world. It gave him a continued sense of purpose, not to mention a paycheck.

"Jerry loved working in the kitchen," Linda Spencer, administrator of the senior center, told me. "You could always hear him laughing and singing. He was always bright and witty. He always tried to be part of things." Linda remembered Jerry as the only person with Alzheimer's she knew who recognized he had Alzheimer's and freely told people about it. "That made a lasting impression on me."

The people at the senior center also showed heartwarming insight and sensitivity in working with Jerry. His coworkers figured out that, as with many people with Alzheimer's, Jerry didn't respond well to spontaneity, so they made sure they didn't spring any surprises on him. In addition, because they knew he was easily rattled, they did what they could to keep him out of the middle of chaos when things got hectic in the kitchen. In this way, they were able to keep Jerry as a productive and beloved member of the kitchen staff for a long time. When it became clear that Jerry was having a hard time keeping up with his kitchen duties, the senior center threw him a big retirement party. Even after Jerry was no longer able to handle his job at the senior center, he continued going there regularly, where he was welcomed by his many friends.

———

It was very sudden and terribly sad when Charlotte became ill. I was stunned at the insight Jerry had into what was happening. He seemed to know and accept that she was going to die. Stephanie dropped Jerry off at the front door of the hospital every day and he usually made it to her room, although after about three weeks, she realized that he was sometimes getting lost in the hospital. Fortunately, he was able to tell someone he was lost.

For a year after Charlotte died, Jerry lived with Stephanie, who was doing her best to figure out how to handle the challenges of caregiving. During this time, we decided to start an intervention group for individuals with young-age-onset Alzheimer's and immediately thought of Jerry.

But because Stephanie was young and busy, it was not feasible for her to bring Jerry to the center for meetings. In order for Jerry to participate, we had to address transportation. We found a trustworthy cab driver to drive Jerry back and forth between his home, Stark Club meetings, and the senior center. Jerry made enormous contributions to the Stark Club. His enthusiasm was a catalyst in winning over some of the more reluctant and skeptical members.

The consistency of having the same driver over the years allowed a relationship to develop between Jerry and the driver. Aware of Jerry's limitations, the driver always made sure Jerry was safe in the house before he drove away. For a time, Jerry and Stephanie did a great job making their arrangement work. It was a while before Jerry needed full-time attention.

And that's when the angel appeared.

———

Joan met Jerry at Sunday school. Jerry, ever the outgoing optimist, set his sights on a date with the attractive blonde.

"He was a neat man, well-mannered," Joan recalls. "He kept wanting my phone number." Joan was cautious and didn't give him her number, but took his. "I thought

I'd call him and tell him, 'Don't call me,'" she says. "I called and he answered the phone. He immediately told me he had Alzheimer's. I'd never been around anyone with Alzheimer's disease before."

Joan agreed to a date. They met at a park, stopped for sandwiches at a nearby sub shop, and then Joan (at Jerry's request) drove Jerry home. "I drove him to the apartment and he said thank you. He was very much a gentleman," Joan says. So when he called again and asked to take her out to dinner (though he said she would have to drive), she said yes.

"Stephanie made sure he had enough money in his billfold to pay for the dinner," Joan recalls. "He was so proud to be with me."

Over time, the two spent increasing time together and the relationship grew deeper. Stephanie was a little skeptical; she didn't really know what Joan's motivations were. Joan's family—a daughter, three sons, fourteen grandchildren and nine great-grandchildren—also weren't sure what to make of the relationship.

But Joan set boundaries and Jerry was a gentleman. Although Joan sometimes wondered if she should marry Jerry, she prayed on the question and got an answer. "The Lord said, 'No, Joan. You're here to be his caregiver, not his wife," she says. "It laid on my heart, too, that Stephanie was young, just twenty-three years old. She had just lost her momma. And she had to take care of Jerry. I just wanted to tell Stephanie to go on with her career, her education, go on with her life and I would take care of Jerry."

And in the end, that's exactly what happened.

In February 2002, Stephanie rented a larger apartment for her and her father. To minimize the stress of the move, with all the boxes and confusion and upheaval, Stephanie and Joan decided that Jerry would stay with Joan for a few weeks until Stephanie had the new apartment in order.

"But he stayed a few more days and a few more days and he didn't come back," Stephanie says.

Jerry was comfortable at Joan's house, he and Joan were exceedingly fond of each other, and the situation just settled itself. "It was clear to us," Joan says.

For Stephanie, this turn of events was a wonderful reprieve. And for Joan and Jerry, the situation just worked. In 2004, Stephanie's company offered her a job in Chicago. With Joan's blessing, Stephanie took the job and moved to Chicago. She continued checking in nightly with her father and visited frequently.

Joan took on the task of day-to-day caregiving with foresight and compassion. She and Jerry created a life for themselves. "Everything just fell into place," she says. Joan's family grew to adore Jerry. "They've all accepted him as family. They love him. When my five-year-old grandson calls, if I answer the phone, he says, 'Let me talk to Jerry.'"

Joan has an almost sixth sense about what Jerry needs, even before she reads about different interventions in books. She learned to draw him out in conversation each evening. "I can prompt," she explains. "I ask, 'What did you do at the senior center, who did you see?'" Even after Jerry was no longer able to express his needs with words, Joan learned to understand him. "If he goes to the kitchen I know he wants a drink of water. If he goes to the hallway, he has to go to the bathroom," she says.

Although many of Jerry's old friends dropped off over time, between the Stark Club, the senior center, church, and Joan and Jerry's families, Joan has made sure Jerry continues enjoying a social life. One year, Joan bought Jerry a Santa outfit he wore for her grandchildren and their friends. "We walked the block and handed out candy canes," Joan says. "Jerry had a lot of fun."

Joan and Jerry enjoy praying and singing together. "At first, when we prayed and the words didn't come out right, he'd get upset that I couldn't understand him. I said, 'Hey, it's all right. The Lord understands. You just say what you want to say.'"

And when Jerry entered Joan in a pageant at the senior center, Joan went to humor him—and won the titles of Miss Congeniality and Miss Mature. Jerry was so proud. He brought photos from the event to the Stark Club to show us all.

Joan was working when Jerry moved in with her, but when he had a seizure at breakfast one morning and fell off a chair, injuring his shoulder, Joan decided it was time for her to retire and care for him full time.

In some ways, Joan says, watching Jerry change as the disease progresses might be easier for her than it would be for a spouse or other family member. "I didn't know Jerry before, as an engineer. I just know this person," she says. "The emotional challenge is different. You're not as emotionally invested."

It's hard not to be awed by a woman like this, who reached out when she saw someone she could help. And it took a huge leap of faith and trust on Stephanie's part to let go, to believe in the goodness of people, to see that allowing Joan to help was not only in her best interest, but even more importantly, in Jerry's best interest. As a young woman alone and on the threshold of adulthood, Stephanie could have provided only so much for a man who would need increasing amounts of support and wisdom as the years passed. Stephanie understood that Joan, at this time in her life, could give that much more.

Joan believes her purpose in life is to be a caregiver. But she also says that Jerry has given back to her as well. Joan's son said it best: "The thing most of us seek in life is simple: to love and be loved. It's hard to find this type of love today. I've found it in Jerry. His love of life, his faith in God, his trust in me, no matter what my shortcomings may be, is unending. The strength and faith I've received through this man is never ending. I will carry it with me the rest of my life."

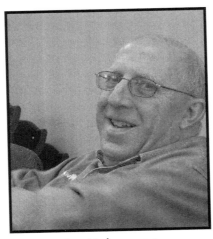

Jay Haberman

Alzheimer's disease didn't rob Jay Haberman of the twinkle in his eyes or his jolly approach to life.

Chapter 3
Facing Down Fear with Fun

"Just keep going and enjoy life."
Jay Haberman

Jay Haberman always has a twinkle in his eye. When he's getting a kick out of something, a mischievous smile creeps over his face and his eyes start dancing. Jay has always considered himself a silly kid.

Unchecked, stress can make life feel out of control, and little is as stressful as a diagnosis of dementia. But Jay's story is about living life with intention, even in the midst of Alzheimer's disease.

Jay is one of those people who has the gift of dealing with whatever life throws his way with a wink and a smile. I guess when you're born with an appreciation of a good joke and a good time, even something as life-changing as Alzheimer's disease isn't enough to completely spoil your fun. That's not to discount the challenges presented along the way, but the combination of Jay's good nature and his wife Frances' bottom-line approach to life have forged a powerful dynamic that has kept them connected to the world around them and the pleasures of life well lived.

I remember once when Jay and Frances were preparing to leave a Stark Club meeting. A group of women were standing by the door, and as he made his way out of the meeting room, Jay insisted on giving every one of them a hug. Because people sometimes undergo changes in their personalities as Alzheimer's progresses, I asked Frances if he'd become more of a hugger since his diagnosis. She rolled her eyes. "Oh no," she said. "He's always been like that." I looked at Jay, who was smiling like the cat that ate the canary. I had to laugh.

Jay's *Collection of Life Stories* book is full of twinkle-in-the-eye humor. One story is about a group of buddies he meets every Thursday to do community projects. They call themselves the Board of Directors. They even have business cards. They do volunteer work and then go out for board lunches, where they "consult with each other about what the waitresses look like," he wrote. Some weeks "we have so much 'business' to discuss that we meet on Tuesdays, too. Our work is just never done!"

The book is full of jolly scenes—Jay cooking traditional potato *latkes* for family and friends at Hanukkah; his fiftieth birthday party; playing "my favorite sport—the slot machines!" on cruise ships. He has a story about catching a big swordfish while deep-sea fishing in Cancun. "Did I mention that Frances went along on this outing?" he wrote. "Did I mention she got seasick?"

Jay and Frances have always had a full and active life. They have two sons, Philip and Adam, lots of friends, and a busy social calendar with dining clubs, activities with their temple, and a love of travel. They have been to France, Spain, Italy, Mexico, and all over the United States.

Jay was in his mid-fifties when Frances noticed he was forgetting words and struggling with such simple activities as ordering his meals in restaurants. And things weren't going well at his job at a cellular phone store.

"They changed to a computerized inventory system and he couldn't do it," Frances recalls. "He was there until 10 p.m. every night. If you didn't get it done fast enough, the computer cut you off. He could never get it done in time."

Jay coped with that problem with his usual geniality. "He just said, 'I'll do it tomorrow,'" Frances recalls. "He didn't take it to heart. He still doesn't, thank goodness."

But, troubled by the struggles she was seeing, Frances insisted Jay see a doctor. I asked Frances how she had persuaded him to do this. Jay, who was sitting silently nearby, piped up with a playful grin and said, "She hits me."

Once Jay sought medical advice, the diagnosis came quickly. A neurologist diagnosed Jay, then fifty-eight, with Alzheimer's. Once they had the diagnosis, Frances and Jay moved forward staunchly. "I wouldn't say it was relief," Frances recalls. "I remember driving around crying and not doing well. I went on Paxil. It was a process to learn how to deal. It was a very traumatic time, obviously. But it just was. There wasn't anything we could do about it."

Jay had lost his job by then (Jay's supervisor told Frances he had been urging Jay to see a doctor for a long time), and the first thing the couple did was consult an elder-law attorney to get their financial affairs in order. This decision was partially motivated by an article Frances read about a woman who only ate peanut butter sandwiches because that was all she could afford. Instead of just worrying about what might happen if they found themselves in a financial crisis, the story prompted Frances and Jay to take action.

"My theory was to take care of the situation and enjoy the life we have," said Frances.

She also found it helpful having an objective third party—a financial advisor—step in when things were still a bit emotional. While a couple has no way to predict the future, "it's good to be prepared and not shocked," Frances advises.

Jay was in the very early stages at that time, and the Habermans were able to make all their preliminary arrangements together. They tried to get long-term care insurance, but when the company called for Jay's qualifying interview, he couldn't answer the questions, and so was denied. Frances, who was able to get long-term coverage for herself, regretted not getting it years ago, when several of their friends had. "We thought we were fine," she says.

And then with all their serious affairs in order, the Habermans chose to continue with life. "I can't sit home all the time, and Jay can't either," Frances says. "I get unhappy if I do. I don't want to think about Alzheimer's all the time. When situations arise, I'll face what I have to."

When a man spoke at their temple about Hearts and Helpers, a volunteer organization that does simple repairs and general handyman work for elderly people, Jay signed up right away. "Jay has always been handy," Frances says. "We didn't have to hire people often."

Jay works with Hearts and Helpers twice a week, and he also works with the Ramp Project a couple of Saturdays each month, building wheelchair ramps for people with disabilities. These projects have been wonderful for Jay, for both the fun and for the satisfaction. "One lady wrote us a thank you note calling us 'the boys,'" he wrote in his *Collection of Life Stories* book. " She was in her eighties, so I guess we were boys to her."

Jay's colleagues at Hearts and Helpers are the same men who comprise the Board of Directors that he wrote about in his *Collection of Life Stories*. Frances is touched by the warmth with which Jay has been supported by the board members, who make sure he always has a ride to and from their "meetings."

Jay also found friends and companionship at the Stark Club, which the Habermans learned about after their evaluation at the center.

Jay really enjoys the camaraderie and joking that goes on in the Stark Club meetings and he consistently finds ways to add to the fun. He often joked about how small the coffee cups were by consistently pouring himself two cups of coffee at every meeting.

"We laugh and cut up a lot," is how Jay describes our meetings. "We have a good time and keep up with new information about Alzheimer's. It's a very supportive group and a fun place to come. The relationships we've formed are wonderful for us both."

Frances, who was still teaching elementary school at the time Jay began coming to the Stark Club, was unable to attend the women's group right away. But about two and a half years after Jay's diagnosis, he passed out in a grocery store as a result of an adjustment in his medication. This event made Frances realize it was time for Jay to stop driving. When she shared her concern with Jay, he agreed to give up the car keys. "I had worried so much about telling Jay not to drive, but most of what I have worried about has never come to pass. Everything happens on its own time scale."

At that time, Frances decided she should retire to spend more time with Jay, and she checked in on the Stark Club women's group, which she found wise and supportive. "We're all in the same boat, and they have helpful things to say," she says. "I remember [another member] telling me that someone had told her, 'Don't project. Just don't project. Live right now.' I think about that."

Frances is otherwise circumspect when it comes to discussing Jay's illness with friends outside the Stark Club, both to spare friends the emotional stress of hearing about it and to take a break from it herself.

"They would empathize and listen, but I don't want them to get bored of listening to me," she says. "I just want to enjoy being with them and not worrying about other things."

When she meets new people, Frances tells them about Jay on a need-to-know basis. "Most people understand if you tell them," she says. "I don't necessarily say anything in front of Jay. If someone asks him a question and he is unable to answer, I will tell people. I used to say he has trouble talking. Now I say he has Alzheimer's."

Frances feels fortunate that she and Jay have been able to continue traveling and socializing. "I've said we were going to do as much as we could as long as we could," Frances says. Sometimes, she admits, she has trouble maintaining the energy and optimism to keep busy and upbeat, but she usually finds it again.

While initially Frances would leave Jay alone for three or four hours at a time, that time has dwindled, mostly because Frances wants to save Jay any worry. "If something does happen—like the time he forgot how to flush the toilet—there's no need for him to be upset for hours until I get back," Frances says.

Board meetings free Frances up for activities she enjoys. Otherwise, rather than curtailing her social life to care for Jay, Frances just brings Jay with her wherever she goes—ladies' movie group, bridge—if it's nothing Jay is interested in and there's a room with a television where he can hang out while Frances visits, he's content.

"Our friends are old friends—we've had them a long time," Frances says. "If I can't bring Jay, I don't go. It's gotten harder, but I feel like I still have my life. If I had to give up activities, then I would be unhappy. Practically, it's worked because I've worked at it. I've been able to help it not overwhelm either one of us."

And they still socialize as a couple. They go to restaurants and Frances knows her husband's tastes well enough to make a few menu suggestions he can choose from. Once, they met another couple at a museum exhibit of Chinese artifacts. They rented earphone tours. "At each numbered marker I helped Jay program his earphones," Frances says. "We just did it the way we always had. It worked great. We both enjoyed the exhibit."

The couple goes to the health club together and Frances sets Jay up on the treadmill or with weight machines while she works out alongside him. And they still travel, with precautions. Once, on a trip to Spain, Jay got up in the middle of the night and walked out of his room looking for Frances. Now she carries an alarm that will sound if Jay gets up in the middle of the night. "So far, I'm the only one who has set it off," she says with a laugh.

Frances still enlists Jay's help in household chores. "Jay always did the yardwork. He always trimmed the shrubs and mowed the yard. He still mows and I tell him how to do the shrubs. On Fridays, we'll go out and work in the backyard together. He hates weeds so he'll pull them up and I'll make sure he doesn't pull out any of my flowers. I keep trying to give him things to do. And household maintenance activities have provided a great activity for Adam and Jay to spend as father and son. He helps me as much as he can. He's not allowed to walk away from the dinner table without clearing his plates."

People who remain tuned in to Jay reap the benefits of his warmth. For example, Jay's friend, Doug Freeman, tells a story about being ordained as a pastor in the Reformed Church in America. "Jay and I do not share the same theological position. Jay is Jewish and I am Christian," Doug wrote in an email. "However, in the days leading up to my ordination on July 25th, Jay continued to make sure that he knew when my ordination service would take place. He continually tried to keep that date alive in his mind. He kept reminding me, but I suspect it was done to remind himself.

"On the day of my ordination service, Jay and his family and friends sat through a lengthy traditional Christian service with Communion. At the end of that service, I was being greeted by many of my friends. As Jay approached there were tears in his eyes, but the words would not come. I finally supplied the words, 'You are proud of me, right?' With a huge sigh of relief, Jay said, 'Yeah!' His greeting and the affection he expressed became a pinnacle moment for me, and one that will be forever remembered."

Frances and Jay haven't let Alzheimer's sideline them, and that's an important lesson. There's no point in living through the future before it even happens. "I know there are changes coming, but I choose not to live in the future," Frances says. "I'm not going through this twice."

Frances feels they have been lucky. Jay's personality has remained as genial and easygoing as ever. "He can't say things he wants to say, but half the time I know what he's going to say," Frances says. And if he's got a twinkle in his eye, he's probably going to say something funny.

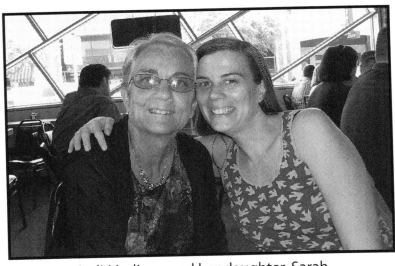

Jodi Madigan and her daughter, Sarah

Creativity is the engine that still drives Jodi Madigan's life despite Primary Progressive Aphasia.

Chapter 4
Bonds Beyond Words

"Never doubt that things will change—they always do. I am confident that things will be better, you will be stronger, life will smile again."
Jodi Madigan

Jodi Madigan was the first woman to join the Stark Club, and when the guys found out she rode a Harley-Davidson, they knew she'd fit right in. Jodi came of age in the tumultuous 1960s. After her boyfriend was killed in Vietnam, she became a peace activist and marched in demonstrations. She also traveled the world and, with her former husband, helped found a restaurant and leather store that became a Dallas institution. Jodi is a gentle hippie soul who loves gardening, making art, and, of course, her children, who have teamed up to help Jodi live the fullest life possible.

In Jodi's world, most things function normally. She cooks her own meals, shops for groceries, keeps up with appointments, and pursues her hobbies of painting, gardening, and photography (to name a few).

What she can't do is talk. At least not like most of us do.

Jodi has Primary Progressive Aphasia (PPA), a disease that gradually degrades a person's ability to talk. Jodi knows what she wants to say, but over time her ability to put her thoughts into words has become more and more difficult.

I've often tried to step into Jodi's world and imagine what life is like for her. I've tried to imagine the frustration of knowing what I want to say but struggling with every word. I've imagined the keen disappointment—as I've often seen on Jodi's face—at failing to clearly communicate a message. And I've imagined the joy of connection that Jodi must feel when, through a combination of pictures, written words on a page, or a series of questions and answers, she successfully relays her message or story.

Jodi's initial challenges with language were much more subtle than what I have just described, but from the very beginning they caused tremendous concern for Jodi and her loved ones about what *might* be happening. In a way, Jodi's diagnosis was a relief to her three children.

For two years, Jodi's ability to communicate had been breaking down. She would mix up the names of her daughters, Claire and Sarah. She made uncharacteristic grammatical errors in her speech. She forgot words—mostly verbs. She mixed up other words.

"Once when we were driving, we got stopped in Arizona and the troopers asked what country we were from. She said 'Texas' and the guys just died laughing," remembers twenty-eight-year-old Sarah, who calls Jodi by the affectionate nickname "Momma Lou."

Jodi, her children, and her boyfriend, Mike, with whom she lived, knew something was wrong, but they didn't know what, and doctors weren't helping much.

"It was two years of different doctors all saying, 'I don't know,'" says her son, Colin.

Some doctors tried to blame menopause. Others (as is so common with early-age dementia) suggested depression.

"Mom has struggled with depression," Sarah acknowledges. "But in the past, it certainly didn't manifest itself this way. It was a cause of a lot of anxiety, but the language problems didn't seem to be symptomatic of anxiety. Some doctors even mentioned the possibility of early Alzheimer's disease, but our grandfather had Alzheimer's disease, and what we remembered of Alzheimer's and what we were seeing didn't match."

Nothing doctors suggested seemed to fit the problems, and not knowing what was happening was terrifying to the family. "We were thinking brain tumor. We were really scared," Sarah says.

The whole family (and Mike was very much part of the family) focused their energy on Jodi's frustrating problem, spending hours online researching communication problems. It was Mike who found a Dallas neurologist specializing in communication disorders. He and Jodi went to see this neurologist, who diagnosed Jodi with Primary Progressive Aphasia.

"I was in the middle of a take-home final exam," recalls Sarah, who was finishing law school in Boston at the time. "I got an email from Mike saying, 'This is what the doctor thinks.' I went to an online medical dictionary and said, 'This is it.' It was the first thing that connected all the dots, that was logical."

After Sarah finished her test (and today she is an attorney, so obviously she somehow managed to stay focused that day), she, Colin, and Claire—who at the time were a tender twenty-five, twenty-three, and twenty-one years old, respectively—got on a conference call together to commiserate and plan.

"We were thankful it wasn't a tumor—something catastrophic and fast," Sarah says. Although Colin adds: "It was a new set of hurdles. It was good to stop the testing and all that, but then we had to start looking for therapies."

For reasons unrelated to PPA, Jodi was out of work at the time of her diagnosis. She had been laid off by a bank well before the diagnosis and had been unable to find another job, although that appeared to be due more to the fact that she was in her fifties than any cognitive difficulties. It is a fascinating aspect of our brains that although Jodi's abilities with words were badly compromised, her facility with numbers was not affected by the disease, and nor was her talent with computers, both skills she used to earn her living. Four years after her diagnosis, Jodi still managed her own finances with no difficulty.

But even before the diagnosis, because of her increasing difficulty communicating, and the frustration of finding a job, Jodi and her children decided that it would be best if she cease her job search and collect disability insurance. "It took us a while to get her insurance and we had to appeal," Sarah says. Fortunately for her and Jodi, the state of Texas recognizes common-law marriages so Mike was able to help in the process. "He sort of finagled and I lawyered," Sarah says.

Meanwhile, the neurologist who diagnosed Jodi recommended the Stark Club to her. Although she would be the first, and at that time, only woman in the group, Jodi immediately joined and became a loyal and avid participant. When Jodi wants to add to a Stark Club discussion, she writes her thoughts and passes them to me to read aloud. Sometimes she comes prepared with pre-written accounts of things she has done, such as when she returned home from a trip visiting Sarah in New York. She brought us pictures and a list of the things they did: Metropolitan Museum of Art, the Guggenheim Art Museum, the Museum of Modern Art, Central Park and Madison Square Park, and a speedboat ride to see the Statue of Liberty.

Because of her limited language, Jodi often needs someone familiar with her life to help her participate fully in Stark Club discussions. Mike, with whom Jodi had been living for four years before the diagnosis, was her primary caregiver, and with his help, Jodi was much more able to participate in Stark Club discussions. For example, one particularly lively and fun activity that requires help from all of the caregivers is a game called "Two Truths and a Lie." At each meeting, one group member comes to group with three statements, one of which is not true. The rest of the Stark Club asks questions and tries to guess which statement is false.

Knowing Jodi's history, Mike helped Jodi create three statements to present to the group: 1) I am a personal friend of Billy Gibbons, guitarist for ZZ Top; 2) I was closely involved in an incident during the civil rights movement that involved U.S. Attorney General Robert Kennedy, and as a result, one of my relatives is mentioned in the movie *Easy Rider*; and 3) When I was in high school, George W. Bush bought me a Coke.

My reaction was an incredulous, "Two of these are true?"

George Bush never bought Jodi a Coke, but her life has been full of amazing adventures. And if you spend even one day with Jodi, you find she is still a do-er.

Jodi's life as a do-er was very evident to me during one of my recent visits to her home. The moment I arrived, Jodi made clear that she needed my words to help her with something. She immediately went to the phone and started dialing a number. She spoke in short phrases then handed me the phone. I had no idea who was on the other end of the line, but I quickly recognized Colin's voice and identified myself. Jodi handed me an email, which I read to Colin, about their plans together that evening. Jodi efficiently helped me to help her.

As supportive as Mike was of Jodi, being the caregiver was difficult. Sarah remembers Mike alluding to the strain of the task, and Sarah started wondering whether they would have to rethink the arrangement. Tragically, they didn't ever have to make that decision. One day, as Mike and Jodi were working together in their garden, Mike had a massive stroke. Jodi ran next door to enlist the neighbor's help calling 911. After a few days in the hospital, Mike passed away. Jodi was devastated. She kept me in the loop on what was happening via email. At Mike's funeral, the Stark Club members arrived in full force to show their support. It meant a great deal to her. It was obvious that Jodi wanted to introduce us all to family and friends, which she accomplished by physically bringing us together. Her presence was all that was necessary to provide the introduction—we were all connected through this fascinating woman. Two years later, the deep sadness of her loss still shows on Jodi's face when she opens her *Collection of Life Stories* book to show me Mike's newspaper obituary.

Now it was entirely up to Sarah, Colin, and Claire to look after Jodi.

Although Jodi functions on a very high level, she and her children knew she could not live alone, and Jodi did not want to move away from Dallas, partly because of the support and camaraderie she enjoyed with the Stark Club.

"People in the Stark Club understand where you're coming from in a different way," Sarah says. "The meetings provide good social interaction and are something mom always looks forward to. We thought it was important to keep that as part of her life."

At this point, their father—Jodi's ex-husband—volunteered to share his home with Jodi. When this came up in a recent discussion of her history, Jodi quickly sketched two rooms with two beds, and showed me the drawing with a pointed look to make sure I understood that this was a completely platonic arrangement. When I asked if she's OK with it, the expression on her face implied she would rather be living elsewhere. The problems that caused their divorce did not magically disappear after the diagnosis, but she was making the best of her new living situation. The arrangement was hard on the kids, too. However, they all agreed that for the time being, it was the best option available to the family.

"He's there, he takes her to the grocery store, they go to the library every Wednesday," Sarah says. "Basically what mom needs is a place to live with an established routine and someone to take her places. He can do it better than any of our lives would permit us to do right now."

I am continually amazed at the children Jodi has raised. Even in their early twenties, all three are mature beyond their years. They work together to provide incredible support and loving care to their mom. "I deal with the money issues and logistics," Sarah says. "Colin deals with the day-to-day stuff, and Claire is the glue that holds us all together."

———

For a long time after the diagnosis, Jodi was able to fill pages and pages of her notebook in making her points to others. She also hung on to a few useful phrases: "Yeah, cool," and "Yes, OK," were among them. Over time, those communication skills eroded and her notes became yet more telegraphic, using series of keywords to get her points across. But as long as people around her stay in tune with her, Jodi lets them know what she needs. For example, when Sarah received an email from Jodi that read, "Jodi check, bank, old address, new address," Sarah gleaned that Jodi needed to go to the bank and get checks with her new address on them. "You definitely get the gist of what she's saying," Sarah says.

In some ways, Jodi's dementia is easier on her loved ones than Alzheimer's disease would be because the aphasia affects verbal communication more than memory and other cognitive processes. While Jodi can't communicate with words, she is not at risk of getting lost, she can enjoy movies, she still takes care of her own physical and many other needs, and she's still the free spirit she has always been. She continues to garden, paint, take pictures, cycle, walk, and travel. While Mike was alive, they continued to enjoy outings on their Harleys. Jodi carefully marks her calendar with details as small as when to change the filter on her water purifier. The area around her computer is a trove of notes and reminders. Her children both watch over her and respect her autonomy.

Every morning, Jodi walks three miles, which she considers the best part of the day. "She carries in her oh-so-stylish fanny pack her name and address, her phone number, my phone number, and a paper that says 'communication problems,'" Sarah says. "Claire and I walk with her when we come home and we can barely keep up," she adds with a laugh. After her walk Jodi tends her beloved garden and birdfeeder.

Sarah and Jodi instant message with each other for about thirty minutes around lunchtime every day, and Sarah uses her camera phone to take and email funny photographs of herself to her mom. "I try to send her a stupid picture every day," she says. When Claire was producing segments for an NPR radio show in San Diego, Jodi emailed every week to learn what Claire was working on, listened to the show online, then sent Claire follow-up emails about her segments and what she liked. "It was really adorable," says Claire, who now works for a newspaper.

Claire and Jodi also email daily and they speak on the phone, although, says Claire, "Phone conversations are pretty rough. I still like to do it every couple of weeks, but I'm leading the conversations. I have to figure out what's going on with her by her limited answers." Clearly, the computer technology that now has become commonplace in our lives has become a blessed lifeline for this close-knit family.

Colin, who lives down the street from his parents, visits several times a week and when Jodi wants to go to Austin to visit old friends, Colin drives her. "I really noticed that when my mom stopped doing things, she got sad," says Colin. "It's good to help keep her busy."

Sarah, Colin, and Claire are very aware of the importance of having something to look forward to and make it a point to always have something on the calendar. Every other weekend Jodi can look forward to a visit from Sarah or Claire, and she continues to make trips to Austin and go out to dinner with friends.

Because Jodi has always been an artist, one of the first things the kids did for her was buy her a digital camera, which she uses avidly. In San Diego, Claire took her to a wildlife park where Jodi took pictures of everything they saw. "She was really excited," Claire says. Of course, those pictures were proudly displayed at the next meeting of the Stark Club.

Jodi also continued painting with watercolors for a long time after her diagnosis. When Sarah noticed that Jodi was not painting as much as she once had, in yet another inspired act of concern, she got back on the Internet and found an art therapist in Dallas to work with Jodi on creative expression of her feelings. The therapist not only helps Jodi remain connected to her creative muse, but also helps her process her grief over Mike's death, which the dementia has prevented her from expressing verbally.

As Jodi's communication skills became further impaired—four years after her diagnosis, she has started mixing up "yes" and "no"—Jodi's children knew they had some difficult decisions ahead of them regarding her living arrangement, and the timing of the move came more quickly than they anticipated. Jodi had been having difficulty walking and was nauseated, so Sarah came home to spend some time with her. Concerned at Jodi's symptoms, Sarah took her to the emergency room where they discovered a bleed on her brain that required emergency surgery. As best as they could determine, Jodi had fallen down the stairs one evening. No one heard her fall, and she chose not to alarm anyone by telling them about the incident. But this caused Jodi's kids to start looking for an assisted living arrangement that would accept Jodi's cats and provide her the option of more activities. The change has been a good one for Jodi. She enjoys having her own space and joining in the activities and outings offered each week.

Despite the stress of looking ahead and the sadness of looking back, Jodi and her children cope with the here and now with love, equanimity, and appreciation. "My mother is still cute and she's still happy," says Claire. "She's very innocent and giggly. Easily amused. If I was her, I don't know how I would have dealt with what happened. There's no way I would have dealt with it as well as she did. I remember her saying, 'If I'm not going to get any better, I'm going to have the best time that I can now.'"

With the support of her family, Jodi is doing exactly that.

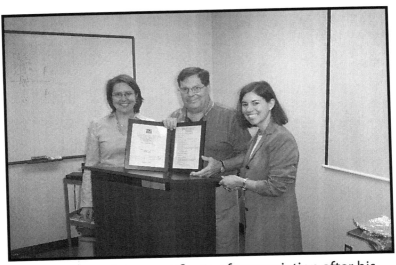

Bill Crist receiving certificate of appreciation after his presentation at the Alzheimer's Association Caregiver Conference.

First Bill was angry about his Lewy body syndrome, then he channeled that energy into helping others.

Chapter 5
From Anger to Activism

*"A lot of people don't know what Alzheimer's is.
One of our roles is to educate people
about Alzheimer's." Bill Crist*

Bill Crist is equal parts tough and tender. He was captain of his high school football team, a Navy flight officer, a competitive runner, an ombudsman at a nursing home, and volunteer companion to a man with Parkinson's. Bill calls things as he sees them, he sees the value in everyone, and he's a man of action— an independent spirit with a talent for leading a team.

When I asked the group how they would describe the Stark Club to someone who had never seen it, Bill's response struck me deeply: "If someone walked in this room right now, we would look like any other mid-life men and women, but with one difference: We have dementia."

So often a diagnosis of dementia causes us to think of all the things a person *can't* do instead of looking for and accentuating things they still *can* do. Bill wants to contribute in life—a desire I believe is held by all people with dementia, especially in the early stage. The sense of contribution is critical for all of us. But when it comes to dementia, we are unknowingly prejudiced, often focusing on the impairments and underestimating what these individuals still can offer.

Yes, change is imminent with progressive dementia, but change happens over time. We need to find acceptance and ways to ease the blow of the diagnosis so individuals can move forward with hope instead of anger. Sometimes, the best person to address issues related to dementia are the people dealing with it.

Bill has Lewy Body disease, but he refers to his diagnosis as Alzheimer's because this is a term people understand. Although his symptoms are different from those of someone with Alzheimer's, he has chosen to use Alzheimer's as a platform to communicate a very important message that hope is powerful medicine.

———

Bill's early symptoms were more physical than cognitive—problems with vision and gross motor skills. He sometimes struggled to clearly express his ideas, sometimes using more words than necessary or using difficult-to-follow syntax. But for the most part, Bill's mind remained sharp and his communication skills were good. He did not fit anyone's mental picture of a man with progressive dementia.

The first symptoms he noticed were flashes of double vision. "It was like a shadow, and when you blink, it's gone," Bill says. Sometimes, he was oddly unable to see things at all. Bill's family initially was more annoyed than concerned. How could they help it? The things Bill was reporting were just—let's face it—weird.

"Once we went to the Monterey Aquarium with our son and daughter-in-law," Bill's wife, Peggy, recalls. "We were in a room with a floor-to-ceiling aquarium. It was a marvelous thing. We were just watching it and Bill said, 'I can't see.' I said, 'What do you mean you can't see?' It was strange and it was annoying. It was so irrational to me that I could not understand it at all, other than to attribute some negative behavioral characteristic to it."

Bill's symptoms were a little bit of this, a little bit of that. They were slow, they were intermittent, they didn't clearly point to anything in particular. With his doctor, Bill talked mostly about his heart and blood pressure so the doctor didn't suspect any neurological problems. And Bill kept struggling along.

But then Bill and Peggy had to drive home to Fort Worth from Maryland the day after the terrorist attacks on New York City and Washington, D.C., in September 2001. For long stretches of the trip, Bill was unable to drive and Peggy had to take the wheel—an unusual situation for the couple. "That's when I knew we had to seek medical help and Bill agreed," Peggy says.

As soon as they got home, and nearly a year after the bizarre experience at the aquarium, the Crists finally laid out all the problems to an internist, who immediately suspected neurological problems. One of the standard neurological tests Bill underwent that day was counting backwards from one hundred by sevens. Although Bill had always been a math whiz, he couldn't do it. The couple made an appointment with a neurologist, who told the couple that Bill had Lewy Body syndrome and bluntly laid out his future—a progressive degeneration of mind and mobility, no more driving a car, no more alcoholic beverages, no more golf.

After all that time of simmering frustration with his situation, this graphic description of the future blew the lid off of Bill's anger. He begged to differ, loudly and emphatically. In fact, he and the neurologist got into a yelling match.

"I was very mad," Bill says, looking back on that stressful day. "Why me? I denied the truth of the results. I was ready for retirement and to play golf. Peggy had her career. From all our planning, we were exactly where we wanted to be. So the diagnosis hit me like a ton of bricks. I couldn't play golf, couldn't drive, couldn't drink. You might as well kill me."

The neurologist was actually following one standard protocol for delivering devastating news: Be firm, be blunt, and don't candy coat anything. This neurologist surely wasn't counting on a strong personality like Bill or the amount of frustration he had built up since the mysterious problems started.

Jennifer took Bill out of the room for a little break and a heartening discussion about the things he still could do despite the disease, and while she was calming him down, she suggested that Bill check out the Stark Club.

"I told Jennifer I'd think about it, but my intention was to go hide somewhere," Bill recalls. Aside from playing team sports, Bill wasn't much of a joiner, but Jennifer didn't give up. She called Bill the day after his diagnosis and left him a message. Bill ignored the call. She called again a day later. Again, he didn't respond. She called a third time the day after that. Finally, ten days after that last call, Bill called her back, and Jennifer managed to persuade him to attend a Stark Club meeting.

Bill being Bill—kind of stubborn, feeling ornery— defied doctor's orders and drove himself to his first Stark Club meeting. He wasn't ready to give up that particular form of independence yet and nobody could make him.

To his surprise, Bill had a great time at the meeting. "Everyone had a genuinely positive attitude," he remembers. "When I first walked in, I hadn't been there ten seconds and this big hulk of a man, Jerry, friendliest guy on the earth, came over, shook my hand and said, 'We're glad you're here.' That's a hard welcome to beat. The group didn't sit around and commiserate; we had meaningful discussions about research on Alzheimer's, current events, politics, and sports."

At that meeting he also met Jack Kalling, another member who lived in Fort Worth. With a smile, Bill recalls that they decided "there was no reason for both of us to break the law, so we decided to carpool to the meetings."

Even though Bill had not completely accepted his diagnosis, committing to the Stark Club was an important leap forward. He still had hope that the whole business of his diagnosis would just go away, but until it did, he was at least ready to approach the new challenge with an open mind.

Bill's early refusal to fully come to terms with the diagnosis was hard on Peggy. She was especially terrified when Bill insisted on driving. Even two of Bill's brothers, both attorneys, were unable to convince Bill of the wisdom of turning over the car keys. "He was intractable about it," Peggy says. "He said, 'I'm going to drive and I'm going to drink.' That caused horrible friction between the two of us. This was all very frightening to me. Not only the financial loss if Bill had an accident, but I knew if Bill hit someone or injured someone, neither of us could live with that."

But Bill had to come to the decision to stop driving in his own time. It did take a scare to convince him; fortunately the consequences were minor. One day, more than a year after his diagnosis, he was driving home through a construction area and lightly sideswiped a piece of construction equipment. When he got home, he turned his car keys over to Peggy.

This may have been the toughest moment for Bill. "Of the decisions that impact your life, that's got to be number one," he says. "Now Peggy has to plan her life around the fact that I can't drive. And that's difficult." Bill looks serious when he says this, but then a wry grin lights his face. "Everyone in the Stark Club feels exactly the same way. In fact, the men all decided that the neurologist was in cahoots with the wives to put the women in power."

In her own way, Peggy was also struggling with the reality of the diagnosis, as well as some shame. As Bill says: "Alzheimer's is not a one-person disease. In our society, the structure the way it is, it's inevitable, it's a husband-and-wife disease, two people, and they might as well both have it because they are both involved in it very deeply."

With tears in her eyes, Peggy confesses, "I didn't want our world disrupted. I wanted him to be healthy. Selfishly, I wanted things to go as we planned." Peggy joined a support group near their home, but all of the men there were caring for elderly parents with Alzheimer's and Peggy didn't feel connected to their problems. She stopped in to the Stark Club spouses' gatherings a couple of times, but at first—still in her own denial—didn't think they could help her. "I didn't think I had anything in common with these women," she says. "Bill was less sick at that time."

But as I've so often seen happen, with time, the reality of Bill's illness sunk in and Peggy realized that the spouses of the Stark Club could share their experience and compassion with her. Eventually, Peggy started attending meetings more regularly and found that she not only had a lot in common with these women, but the rapport they all developed was a lifeline for her. "We talk about some very frank topics, very personal things," she says, adding that nobody understands the nuances of living with a partner with dementia better than others facing similar challenges. "I have friends I'm very close to outside of the group, but hard as they try, they don't have the empathy or full understanding that the group does."

Both Bill and Peggy learned that a rough road is a lot smoother in the company of kindred spirits. This was the beginning of the end of their anger and helplessness. By taking action in their own lives to adapt to the situation, Peggy and Bill found their footing and Bill took his first step toward speaking out on a larger platform.

Nevertheless, Bill still chose to be private about his illness. Maybe he somehow bought into the dementia stereotypes. Or maybe he feared he couldn't change people's minds if they believed those stereotypes. He kept his condition a secret from neighbors for as long as he could. "He was even embarrassed at first when he started to use the Handitran (public transportation for people with disabilities)," says Peggy. "We were open with the family, but less so with friends. People would ask me at parties if Bill was OK and I would say, 'Of course he is,' and glare at them."

Bill told his golfing buddies, but consistently chooses not to dwell on it with other people. His friends respect him and give him that space. "Bill's dementia has appeared to his friends as a fairly gradual, physically debilitating disease," says Spence Tucker, a friend of thirty years. "I should note that his friends aren't getting any younger either—in most ways Bill just seems to be on an accelerated pace."

Meanwhile, Bill became an important leader within the Stark Club. He's one of the group's deep thinkers. Bill values education and has now expanded his topics of interest to include learning more about Lewy Body disease. He quickly discovered that most news articles were about Alzheimer's, but immediately began learning what he could and shared his new found knowledge.

Realizing a first-person viewpoint of dementia was missing from these articles, the Stark Club decided to create a newsletter with members' personal perspectives and knowledge of dementia. In line with their positive outlook, members chose to title the newsletter, *The Good News about Bad News*. The newsletter addressed such topics as the differences in types of dementia, and how hope and purpose can continue after a diagnosis. And in the newsletter, Bill ranked joining the Stark Club as one of the most beneficial things that happened since his diagnosis. He said, "It is good to have a place to go when you're down, but we never focus on discouraging things. I always learn something and leave feeling better for time spent."

Realizing the value of the meetings to all of the group members, Bill grew involved in ensuring the group stays on the most beneficial track for all members, including the caregivers. He sometimes phones me with suggestions or concerns. From these calls, I've gotten a taste of what a wonderful boss Bill must have been. Once, he thought I might be making a decision that would be detrimental to the group's dynamics and called to discuss it with me. He was so diplomatic, thoughtful, and gentle, I could only be moved and appreciative of his concern and initiative. We talked through the matter and realized that he had misunderstood my intentions. I got off the phone feeling great about being on the Stark Club team with someone who cares and thinks so deeply.

These qualities make Bill an extraordinary spokesman for people with dementia. At the center we often recommend Bill to journalists and others who approach us looking for spokespeople. In 2005, Bill and Peggy were interviewed by an Associated Press reporter about the importance of screening for dementia, and he gave a presentation to a meeting of the North Central Texas Chapter of the Alzheimer's Association in which he proved that nobody can discuss dementia more effectively than someone who speaks of it firsthand.

Just as Bill knows where he stands on politics and current events, he had a definite idea of what he wanted to communicate in his presentation and needed little help. At the next Stark Club meeting, Jennifer and I presented Bill with a Certificate of Appreciation and a list of the many glowing comments from conference attendees. We also played an audio tape of Bill's portion of the presentation for the group, which erupted in applause at the end. It was then I learned that Bill had *thought* he would be speaking to a small breakout group. "I didn't know I would be speaking to five hundred people," Bill said.

Reaching out to people and presenting the strong, capable, human face of dementia to the world is now deeply meaningful and important to Bill, who keeps the Certificate of Appreciation on his mantel at home as a reminder that he is making a difference in the world.

Bill is still Bill. Like any proud granddad, he beams as he shares photos of his brand new granddaughter with his friends at a Stark Club meeting. Although vision problems interfere with his ability to read, he still listens to books on tape from the free Library of Congress service. And, Peggy says, he still can be an ornery political beast. "There's a big friction in our life called Fox News," she says with a laugh. "It is on from the time I get home until I go to bed."

But in a way, that's a good kind of friction. It means despite everything, Bill is still one smart, tough, ornery, loving, intellectual, insightful guy.

"My favorite quote is, 'Let's get the hell out of here,'" says Bill. "Today it takes on a whole new meaning. For me, it means taking my condition and giving everything I've got to fight this battle and leave the negative behind. Thanks to my dear friends and family, I've been given the strength and love needed to persevere. And for that, I'm grateful."

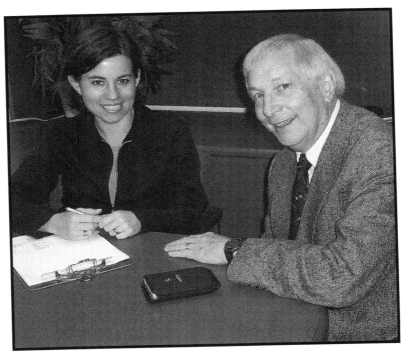

Robert Eshbaugh

Semantic dementia is difficult to diagnose, but once Bob Eshbaugh knew what he faced, he did so with grace and charm.

Chapter 6
Decoding the Truth about Dementia

"Just move on." Robert Eshbaugh

As a successful broadcast engineer in the television news business, including many years with NBC, Robert Eshbaugh spent his life chasing excitement. He was in Mexico for Pope John Paul II's first visit in 1979, was witness to the unrest in Panama in the early 1980s, and he covered the aftermath of the huge earthquake in Mexico City in 1985, working with Tom Brokaw. Robert was often the instigator of boyish hijinx among his colleagues, and with a mischievous twinkle in his eyes, he had a witty catchphrase for everything: "We work hard, we play hard!" and "Get out of our way, we're the wave of the future!"

We all take for granted being able to name everyday things such as a car, a telephone, or a purse, and even less common objects such as a tractor, tape recorder, or bankcard. But what if you started having trouble naming objects—even when given clues, such as "it is has numbers and is used to tell time?"

Normally, you would immediately guess a "clock" or "watch," but this kind of simple information can disintegrate with Semantic dementia, a disease that causes the neural connections between features of an object and the name of the object to malfunction. To add to the confusion, people with Semantic dementia can still use the objects normally—at least in the early disease stages. For some years, people with Semantic dementia seem normal in almost every other way. Their memories remain strong, they still can drive, and can even balance a checkbook. Imagine how frightening and confusing it is to function perfectly in so many ways, but imperfectly in one such important way—and to have no idea why.

I met Robert and his wife, Marie, during their two-year search for a diagnosis of the problems Robert had been having with communication. Initially, a neurologist had diagnosed Robert with depression, but after months of treatment with no improvement, the Eshbaughs sought a second opinion. This time the neurologist suggested that Robert might have either Alzheimer's or Pick's disease— a form of dementia that causes particularly distressing changes, such as vulgar and inappropriate behavior.

At the neurologist's suggestion, the Eshbaughs came to see the specialized diagnostic team at the Alzheimer's Disease Center at The University of Texas Southwestern Medical Center. The Center for BrainHealth was part of that team and would provide in-depth language and cognitive testing.

While Robert was being evaluated, I sat down with Marie to learn about their daily challenges. My heart immediately went out to her. Something was wrong and they needed answers. She was obviously angry with Robert and frustrated with herself. Tensions between the couple were at an all-time high.

Marie told me how Robert had started a new job and just couldn't settle in: "He comes home at night like a zombie—totally exhausted and beat down. He seems paranoid." Marie felt Robert was being intentionally difficult and that infuriated her. She had a hard time reconciling the fact that Robert could still do a lot of things—surf the Web, make music CDs, and do electric repairs on their home— but he couldn't carry on a conversation. Robert could still drive, but couldn't give directions. Marie also confessed that her friends accused her of being too hard on Robert. But she would tell him things he would later claim she had never told him.

"Our conversations consisted of, 'I already told you that.' 'No, you didn't.' 'Yes, I did.' 'Why don't you ever listen to me?'" Marie says. "He doesn't make sense and he won't give me the floor. It's driving me crazy! I can only imagine how it is for people at work. He is short-tempered. He gets so upset he pounds on the table and grits his teeth, and it is often over nothing. This behavior is so out of character for Robert."

Meanwhile in the testing room, Robert was complaining to my colleague, Jennifer, about Marie's impatience. "Why is she yelling at me when I'm trying so hard?" he said. "She's mad and I don't give a damn."

In his testing, Robert soon proved to us that he didn't have memory problems. Semantic dementia is often misdiagnosed as Alzheimer's, which is a disease that primarily affects memory. But it was clear that any information Robert understood, he could remember. What he struggled with was understanding, or "encoding," the information. When we made this crucial distinction, we were able to reach the diagnosis of Semantic dementia. Robert was sixty-one years old.

———

We can all identify with word-finding problems, but the language difficulties associated with Semantic dementia are much different. People with Semantic dementia gradually lose the meaning of words. For Robert, people became pronouns, and he quit calling things by their names (a person with Semantic dementia might say "fluid" or "stuff" to mean "milk"). Robert could string words together and it was clear he had something specific to say, but what? Sometimes, he would use hundreds and hundreds of words in his effort to be understood. He would overwhelm friends with the sheer volume of words, and they would pretend to understand what he was saying. Asking questions to try and decode the message only added another layer of difficulty. Not only did Robert have difficulty getting his message across, he had difficulty understanding what others said to him.

In our treatment program, Robert learned strategies to help him communicate. One strategy was carrying a card in his wallet to show people when he was having difficulty communicating. Printed on the card were the words "I have a language problem. Please be patient with me." This strategy fit perfectly with Robert's can-do attitude.

As time passed, Robert's difficulty with language increased. One of Marie's biggest fears was that Robert would completely lose his connection to people. She had already noticed him pulling away during social occasions. "People tend to talk around him," she lamented to me once. "It's like he's becoming an object in the room."

I have seen a number of people who suffer from Semantic dementia over the years, and I was heartsick to see someone as young and productive as Robert with it. But with a clear diagnosis and the stimulation and support of the Stark Club, I saw Robert change from an angry, fearful individual to one with a strong will to live and a new mission to spread happiness, even in the progressive march of a brain disease that strips people of their nouns and verbs.

Robert found a renewed energy for life and busied himself in new activities, including a research treatment program at the Center for BrainHealth. The research program brought Robert to the center on a weekly basis and he never arrived empty-handed. He brought gifts of music CDs he burned for us. With sparkling eyes and his arresting smile he would say, "I just wanted to cheer you up for doing so much," and then pass out copies of his newest musical compilation to everyone in the office. The CDs were full of cheerful music. What impressed me about Robert was that he was the one who had just received a challenging diagnosis and here he was, coming to cheer up our office.

By this time, Robert had been part of the Stark Club for a couple of years, but Marie had not been part of that group interaction. One of the first times Marie saw Robert in a social environment outside of their own circle was at a Stark Club-hosted event for family and friends of people with Alzheimer's disease and other dementias. Marie remembers that day as the first time she had seen Robert interact in a long time. "It did my heart good to see that side of him in action once again," she says. Instead of just being an observer, Robert was an active participant in t he socializing, , even though his previous volume of words was now replaced with a repertoire of vague phrases: "Only in America," "Just move on," and "You got that right." They were stock expressions, but nevertheless served to connect him to the conversation.

For example, when asked what he thought about the crowd of people at the event, Robert replied, "Only in America." When handing door prizes to winners, he congratulated them with a smile and an encouraging, "Only in America." If he wanted to communicate something but had difficulty getting his message across, he would pause, smile, and make a graceful exit with "Only in America." This phrase became Robert's trademark in the Stark Club. In fact, when Bill Tuel found a Kleenex box with an American flag on it, he bought it for Robert as a gift and it immediately became a beloved possession.

Another beloved possession gained from Robert's participation in the Stark Club is his *Collection of Life Stories*. Working with Robert to record his stories and pair them with pictures was a wonderful experience. Now, with his book in hand, Robert does not have to struggle to introduce a topic—he can just open the book and point to a picture paired with a personal story. While others read the story, he can laugh and say, "You got that right," or "Only in America."

"The book allows him to communicate and connect with people who don't even know him," says Marie happily. "When we have friends come visit, if they haven't been here in a while, we all sit on the couch and read it. The stories can fill in for Robert where the words leave off and give him a new way to connect.

As anyone caring for a person with dementia knows, the road can be lonely. People coping with Semantic dementia have a particular challenge in this respect because the disease often causes affected individuals to lose the ability to empathize. Robert had always been very considerate of Marie, so she was understandably hurt when he started acting insensitively—sometimes refusing to help her with small chores when she asked, for example.

"He would wrinkle up his mouth and look at me like I was Cruella DeVille," Marie says. But when Marie came to understand this as a symptom of the disease, she accepted it. And she appreciates all the more the other ways Robert still shows his affection. "If he hears me in the kitchen, he'll join me there," she says. "He is attentive to helping around the house by setting the table for meals or getting drinks out of the refrigerator. He still prepares the coffee each night, putting the coffee maker on delayed brew, for the next morning. And he helps me keep track of important tasks, although he sometimes needs my help to interpret his communication. Yesterday he wanted me to put gas in the car. At first I could not figure out what he wanted me to do. Finally, he went to the car and I understood. He knew we needed gas."

Robert also likes Marie to join him in front of the television in the evenings. He remains loyal to NBC news and watches it every evening. As they watch, he'll look over at her and his smile speaks of his love and appreciation for her company.

Sometimes as people with Semantic dementia lose the ability to communicate in one way, another way emerges in a fascinating turn of events. Seemingly out of nowhere, and as never before, Robert suddenly could draw. His drawings were beautiful and incredibly precise. We used his newfound talent to make Stark Club greeting cards for various occasions. When the group adopted a soldier who was serving in Iraq, our care packages always included a card from the group that Robert had drawn.

Creativity has become a hallmark of living with Semantic dementia: facing fear with a positive, hopeful response to challenges. Robert would be the first to admit that the decision to stop driving was not an easy one, especially when it necessitated selling his beloved Jeep. But capitalizing on his optimistic attitude and intact "tinkering" abilities, he resurrected a discarded bicycle he found in the alley on trash day and began riding all over the neighborhood. "Robert really has enjoyed that bike," Marie laughs. She also feels it was a moment that told her he had come to terms with his diagnosis and was ready to, as he liked to say, just move on.

Like many forms of dementia, Semantic dementia is a progressive disease, which means caregivers must be flexible and ready for change while remaining sensitive to the needs of the affected individual. When maintaining the home the couple lived in for twenty-five years became difficult and stressful for Marie, her initial talk about moving into an easier-to-maintain apartment was met with resistance from Robert. At that time, Robert was still able to communicate in words—and did. "He said, 'I don't care what you do, I'm not moving,'" Marie recalls. Although Marie was ready to move, she knew she would be wiser to wait before taking on this necessary but disruptive change. A full year passed.

By the time the Eshbaughs did start looking at apartments, Robert's language skills had become more impaired, but he still was able to participate in the decision through facial and nonverbal expression. "There were several apartments we looked at that made him really forlorn, he was shaking his head," says Marie. "I knew he wanted something light and bright and a little newer. He didn't want to settle for less." And so Marie, sensitive to the messages Robert was sending, continued the search. "We finally found a gated community that was most acceptable to him." Robert was still uneasy about the move, but Marie was confident she had made the decision with sensitivity to his needs and desires.

Nevertheless, as with all dementia patients who rely on routine and predictability to feel secure, the process of moving was difficult for Robert. When the young man who had purchased some of the Eshbaughs' family room furniture picked it up, Robert helped load it all into the van. But then when he returned to finish the DVD he'd been watching earlier, he was confused by the emptied room. "He looked around and was so perplexed," Marie says. "I feathered his nest a little with what was left and he was a bit more at peace with it all."

As Robert and Marie have experienced, the importance of routine and predictability in the lives of people with dementia cannot be overstated. Presumably, routines are soothing to people for whom so much has changed and become incomprehensible, even though for their loved ones this can be both difficult to maintain (as in the necessity of moving) and sometimes surprising. For example, Robert watches the same DVDs over and over for hours and hours. Knowing this, his son Jeff sent him a collection of Steve McQueen DVDs for Father's Day. But because the story lines of the movies he had already watched many times were ingrained in Robert's mind, allowing him to follow and understand them even after the disease's onset, the old movies were much more appealing to him than anything new. For Robert, watching a new movie is comparable to someone without the disease watching a foreign-language film with no subtitles.

"He opened [the movies], put one in and took it out, mumbled about something, then put it in the garage sale pile," Marie says. "He tried to give it to (Stark Club friend) Tom Keppler. Finally, he gave it to the young fellow who bought the couch. Now it's gone, and he's happy."

However, change can be positive for people with dementia. After the Eshbaughs lived in their new home for a while, they decided to build a home in a gated community where they would be neighbors with two other Stark Club couples. This close proximity of members is a wonderful development. It means the care-giving wives can support each other while the men with dementia will have nearby friends. And this is a good long-term decision for Marie.

"It's important to try to have a life at the same time as taking care of the present, otherwise you go crazy," Marie says. "None of us knows what tomorrow brings, whether you're healthy or not. It's important to live each day and bring good things into your life."

And Marie is always looking for ways to bring good things into Robert's life. Because he likes having things to look forward to, Marie gives Robert daily updates on activities and events that are coming up. Robert likes going to the grocery store with Marie and always remembers when they need to restock on ice cream. A friend whose husband passed away from Alzheimer's disease sometimes stops by to take Robert to lunch at Wendy's (one of his favorite places) or to a movie. And on Thursdays, Marie and Robert go to a nearby senior center for lunch and to listen to Big Band music, sometimes meeting other couples from the Stark Club there.

With a life as thrilling as Robert's was before Semantic dementia, his *Collection of Life Stories* book is full of grand adventures and great stories, and he loves to relive and share them with friends and loved ones.

Robert would tell you that life is not about feeling sorry for yourself. Just move on and focus your efforts on what you can do, not on what you can't do. His life chasing excitement in the television news business was good training for Robert and Marie, as they break free of the bondage of fear that was hurting their marriage and move forward with their life together.

"I won't deny that living with dementia has changed our lives in many ways," says Marie, "but we have both gained a new perspective. And with the support of the Stark Club, Robert has discovered that he is still the same person he has always been."

Most nouns and verbs are completely gone from Robert's conversations. He speaks only in pat phrases now, but says more with those few words and his big smile than most of us say with thousands of fancy words. Deep inside his brain, the organization and retrieval of words has been destroyed, but not Robert's integrity or compassion or purpose. He lives in a way that has diminished the fear and caused him to discover the courage to continue pursuing life.

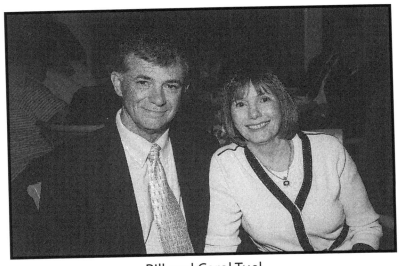

Bill and Carol Tuel

When Bill Tuel finally admitted the troubles Alzheimer's was causing him, he reclaimed his place as pillar of his family.

Chapter 7
Reclaiming Wholeness
from Despair

*"Don't be in denial about changes in yourself.
Don't be ashamed to ask for help." Bill Tuel*

From the time he was a young boy, Bill Tuel was a caretaker—the reliable one, the responsible one, the protector, and the go-to guy to keep things together. He started contributing financially to his family at the age of twelve, and this rock-of-Gibraltar approach to life continued through a distinguished Navy career (where his commanding officer dubbed him "Cool Tuel"), into his pioneering career in computer integration, and to his most treasured job, as father of six.

Employers don't typically expect a disease such as Alzheimer's to strike workers who are only fifty or sixty years old. Poor work performance is among the first indicators of a problem with dementia, but managers may not recognize the signs, both because it is unexpected and because individuals develop sophisticated ways of hiding their struggles.

When job performance continues declining, supervisors usually see no choice but to terminate employment. From that point, without a clear diagnosis and proper documentation, families are in a race with time to qualify for long-term disability—and they may not even know it. Finding doctors and other professionals with specific experience with dementia and the willingness to help with the documentation necessary to qualify for disability is critical for families.

However, back at home, families often don't even realize the extent of the problems happening in the dementia sufferer's workplace until it's almost too late. That is what happened to Bill and his wife, Carol.

Bill knows people look to him to keep things together, and he's always taken great joy in providing financially and emotionally for his loved ones. So when he realized that he was having trouble keeping himself together, he kept his fears to himself. He was having memory lapses, his thoughts were getting scrambled, and he was struggling at his job. But he didn't know how to break the news to his wife, Carol.

The couple was at a financially demanding time in their lives, with the last two of their six children in college. Carol, a homemaker, was accustomed to letting Bill handle many of the logistics of their lives, from bills to home repairs. Although she noticed some memory lapses—for example, he regularly would leave for work and soon return home because he'd forgotten something—she was initially more annoyed than concerned. The problems at home were small, and she had no clue about the difficulties Bill was having at work.

"I didn't even know what Bill did at work," Carol confesses. "He had his work and then he had his life at home with us. I honestly had no clue what he did all day. Looking back, if I had known, I would have had more of an idea of what was going on.

"At first, I thought his symptoms might be attributable to diabetes because his memory lapses coincided with a diagnosis of Type II diabetes. Diabetes became the big focus in our life. We changed the way Bill ate, he lost seventy pounds, we started testing his blood. Then we went home to California to visit my family and they were shocked. They started asking Bill, 'How are you doing at work?' He would say, 'I'm doing fine at work. Everything's fine.' But he had started coming home and falling asleep immediately. I'd say, 'I don't see how you can be doing fine at work when you're like this at home.'"

Nearly two years after Bill's symptoms began, they mentioned his cognitive problems to his endocrinologist, assuming they were associated with the diabetes. Carol recalls, "When the endocrinologist heard Bill's symptoms, he seemed startled. He told us that none of his other diabetes patients exhibited such symptoms and urged Bill to get a neurological exam. We immediately called a neurologist, but the earliest available appointment was August 25, three months away."

At that point, the clock started ticking for the Tuels. Every day counted, as time ran out on Bill's employment, and their window of opportunity to file for his disability insurance edged close. Every day mattered—even more than Carol realized at the time.

On August 8, Bill's employer gave him thirty days to find another job within the company or he would be terminated. Bill had been getting up at 3 a.m. to go to work just to try to keep up, and this on-the-job lapses had become increasingly apparent to his employer. That day, Bill signed a termination letter without understanding its content. A termination would disqualify Bill for disability. Bill did not grasp the enormity of the situation, and he did not even mention it to Carol.

———

More than a week later, Carol still had no idea about the termination letter, but she started to realize something was seriously awry with Bill's work situation.

"Bill was upstairs on the computer. He used to use the computer at home all the time, but he never did that anymore," she remembers. "He was sitting there and for the first time, I was watching him. He could not type. I said, 'What are you doing?' He said, 'I have to update my resume.' The company was having problems at that time and I assumed it was due to that. But nothing made sense about what he was typing."

At that moment, both Carol and Bill understood that things had to change.

"I said, 'Bill, this is it. You cannot go back to work. It's over,'" Carol recalls.

"It was a relief when she said that," Bill says. Finally, at age sixty, he was ready to share the burden he had carried alone for two long years.

The next day, Carol went to Bill's office and they signed on to his work system to research his benefits and how they needed to proceed to file for them.

"His memory was so bad, I felt we needed to file for short-term disability," Carol recalls. "The first step in filing for disability was to contact his manager. Bill couldn't remember what he needed to say, so I had to write down exactly what he needed to ask his manager. I listened in on the conversation and remember feeling his manager sounded very troubled. I knew something wasn't right."

In the following days, Bill continued trying to update his resumé on the home computer, without success. Then, the long-awaited appointment with the neurologist brought a stunning diagnosis: Alzheimer's disease.

As frightening as the diagnosis was, at least it finally shed light on the confusing problems Bill had been having. However, Carol was puzzled by his continuing efforts to update his resumé, so she decided a trip to his office was warranted to see if his desk held any new information.

What she found at Bill's office shocked her.

"His office was plastered in post-it notes," she recalls. Bill's office had recently upgraded their computer operating system and, although Bill was a computer professional, he had struggled with the change. To help him, loyal co-workers had made notes and cheat sheets that were posted all around his computer.

"Since I worked in a technical area, a lot of the problems I was having were compounded," Bill says. He not only struggled with the content of his job, but even with the tools of it.

Yet more distressing, Carol also found the letter Bill signed with a termination date of September 8—now just over a week away.

"When I asked Bill about it, he was under the impression the letter meant he was going to be moved to another job," she says. "He had no idea he had been fired."

Finally Carol had gained as much insight into the severity of Bill's problems as his manager and co-workers, but she was afraid it was too late. A few days later, the disability office called and informed the Tuels that Bill's request for short-term disability had been denied. A diagnosis alone was insufficient for the insurance company. They required specific information to verify Bill's inability to perform the functions of his job.

At this point, the Tuels' nightmare got worse. Although Bill's problems were evident and his neurological evaluation resulted in the diagnosis of Alzheimer's, their neurologist pled ignorance when it came to helping them file for the disability benefits that would keep them financially solvent. Carol and Bill had fifteen days to provide the necessary information to the insurance company and didn't know how to do it or where to start. Carol—who had never even paid the family bills—suddenly found herself in a struggle with the insurance company.

"Some kind of adrenaline kicked in," Carol says. "If I get backed into a corner, I don't take it easily. I learned that if a person is terminated for poor performance, they are no longer entitled for long-term disability. When I realized that Bill might not get the long-term disability that he paid for, I got angry. If I think there's been an injustice, I have a very hard time sitting still for it."

Carol was given the runaround by people at the insurance company, who were skeptical of her claims. "I felt like everywhere I went, I needed to apologize, that it was this shameful thing," Carol says. "Bill had paid for long-term disability benefits, but they made me feel like I was applying for welfare. Our insurance company caseworkers seemed suspicious and said things like, 'Oh, you think your husband has memory loss. Well, I have memory loss if I don't have my morning coffee.'"

In addition, the Tuels had trouble learning the criteria the insurance company used to determine disability. "Part of the problem was that most people think of Alzheimer's as an old-person's disease and Bill was relatively young. People wanted to shrug Bill's problem off as stress, depression, or problems at home," Carol says. "It seemed no one believed me and we were running out of time."

Carol's stress level was at an all-time high, and she felt at the mercy of the insurance company.

"This was the time I needed to be strong and on top of everything and I felt the least strong and the most vulnerable," remembers Carol.""So I did two things: I hired a lawyer and searched the Internet. I was at my wits end when I found the Center for BrainHealth on the Internet. I called and spoke with Jennifer. She patiently listened to my story and immediately said, 'We can help.' I felt myself relax for the first time. No words could have been more welcome. Instead of my begging for help, someone was actually offering help. For the first time, we felt hope.

"Being able to confirm to the insurance company that we found a place to complete more thorough testing satisfied them and we got a little more breathing room; a thirty-day appeal was granted. On the advice of our attorney, I proceeded to make an appointment with a second neurologist to be certain our bases were covered."

With the evaluation in hand, Jennifer worked with the Tuels' attorney to secure Bill's benefits. Within eight days of their coming to the center, Bill had his short-term disability benefits. The long-term benefits followed, although those require periodic re-filing, which Carol continues to manage.

The Tuels' story speaks to the multitude of issues families deal with, not only in getting a diagnosis, but also in adjusting their lives to a frightening new reality. While families do want to know more about the disease, they already are overwhelmed and struggling to find the energy necessary to sort through the volumes of information on Alzheimer's disease.

One focus of the center is to help people get on a positive track early in the disease process and the Stark Club is part of that process. Bill and Carol were pleased to learn of the Stark Club and readily became committed members.

In addition to getting involved in the Stark Club, Bill looked for other ways to contribute. One thing immediately stood out to Bill about his evaluation: "Jennifer told me one of my strengths is reading," he reports. So, for the past two years, Bill has volunteered at a Head Start class several days a week. During playtime, children pick out a book and bring it to Bill to read. Carol was concerned about how parents would respond to Bill working with their children if they knew he had Alzheimer's disease, but that worry was unfounded—Bill was nominated by the City of McKinney, Texas, for Volunteer of the Year.

Problem solving and high-level thinking have always been among Bill's greatest strengths. His job as a solutions architect for a Fortune 500 firm was all about problem solving, generating ideas, and coming up with concepts. Bill is organized and logical and those traits, for the most part, remained intact once the disease started its creep, even if he has more trouble expressing his ideas. He often gets lost between starting to articulate a thought and completing it, but with a little nudge, a little structure, he eventually finds his way back on track.

If friends and family provide a sort of "scaffolding"—a structure of thought to help support, direct, and bolster the ideas a person is trying to express—people in early and mid-stages of Alzheimer's disease can often communicate fairly complex ideas.

Bill and Carol make a remarkable team in that way. Carol seems to instinctively know when to help and when to hold back. The scaffolding Carol provides might mean rephrasing or repeating a question. Sometimes Bill needs help finding a word. When the Tuels joined Jennifer, Sandi and me in making a presentation about Alzheimer's to hundreds of people at the Southwest Dental Conference, Bill did a great job communicating his personal story with the help of gentle reminders or questions from Carol when he needed to be steered back to his point.

And not only does Carol know how to help, but their children still consider Bill the sage of the Tuel family.

Their children call frequently, seeking their parents' guidance. "If they get into too complicated a conversation, Bill turns the phone over to me," Carol says. "He can still comprehend the kinds of circumstances they're in, even if he can't totally articulate it. Sometimes he'll have me write down things he wants me to say to them. And he'll still cut to the bottom line if he thinks they're being immature or not handling things right."

What Bill did lose quickly were his nonverbal problem-solving skills. This meant, for example, that driving was immediately out of the question (as it is for all people with Alzheimer's disease—a change that is often as devastating for them as the diagnosis itself). Carol took over all the driving, although Bill still sometimes can help with navigation. The Tuels also decided to sell their home and move into an apartment because Bill was no longer able to make home repairs or do yard work. Moving to a lower-maintenance home removed a tremendous stressor from their lives. In addition, says Carol, it was a moment of acceptance that their lives had changed.

"It's not really helpful to try to pretend that things aren't the way they really are," she says. "I realized that staying in our big house with the yard and the pool would be like pretending that our life hasn't drastically changed, and it has. That was important for the kids to understand, too."

While acceptance and realism are important in order to make sensible adaptations, this doesn't mean that families touched by dementia should give up all the things they love. About two years after Bill's diagnosis, the couple and three of their sons took a vacation to England and Ireland—a gift to Bill and Carol from all their children. On the trip, Bill was fully able to enjoy and appreciate museums and historical sites. "My long-term memory is full of everything," he says with a wry grin.

However, the family did have to adapt to his deficits in nonverbal problem solving and sequential processes. For example, Bill had problems using the turnstiles in London's Tube, but this was easy enough to work around. "I would buy the ticket and I would hand Bill his," Carol explains. "Right away, the boys figured out that dad had to be in the middle of us. And they started keeping score. After he did it right two out of five times, they said let's see if you can get five out of five today. On the last day, he did get five out of five."

In addition, Carol says, to make sure they could keep track of Bill on the trip, he wore a red ball cap at all times. "I counted and there were only two men in all of London that had on ball caps and Bill was one of them," Carol says with a laugh. "Plus, he was the tallest person in London."

Of course, things did go awry from time to time. Although it was scary at the time, Bill now laughs about getting locked in the airplane restroom in the middle of the night on the way to Europe while Carol and his sons slept. "One of the things that I struggle with is cognitive things, and it became very clear on that flight," Bill says. The complication of having to slide the bolt and turn the handle was too much for him. "I started hollering, 'Somebody PLEASE come open this door,'" he says with a chuckle. Eventually, a flight attendant freed him and helped him find his way back to his seat row—where Carol was still sleeping peacefully. Bill was none the worse for it and had a good story to tell on himself when he got home.

"He jokes a lot about the mistakes he makes," Carol says. "If you never talk about the challenges you face, people may assume you are feeling sad and awful and avoid the topic altogether."

"Bill calls us often and he loves to share some funny story about himself and his latest Alzheimer's disease mishap, finding humor in his present situation," says Carol's mother, Frances Reilly, with whom Bill has always shared a very close relationship (as well as with his father-in-law, Tom).

This is a good lesson and one that some people learn more easily than others. While some individuals try to hide dementia from the outside world, others seem to instinctively understand that other people will follow their lead. Openness can help educate others about the disease, reduce the stigma associated with it, and free the person with the diagnosis to enjoy life rather than focus energy on keeping their diagnosis a secret. As Bill once said: "Why would anyone want to keep a diagnosis a secret? People are going to find out sooner or later."

When Bill was first diagnosed, some casual friends pulled away from the family, although close friends were as devastated as the family and rallied around them. "We realized it helped people to be up-front about the diagnosis," says Carol. "It helps them to feel comfortable with us and ask questions." A former pastor advised Carol not to speak negatively about their situation and just to have faith and it would go away—and Carol immediately scratched him off their list of intimates.

The Tuels' children continue giving back to their father as much as he gave to them over the years. Steve, an accountant who had been living in Michigan, immediately returned to Texas, in large part because he wanted to be near his parents.

There was, of course, an emotional adjustment for the children. Bill, Jr., says his first reaction was anger. "Here was a man who devoted his entire life to God and family and this is how he is thanked?"

And the trip to Europe was an eye opener for Matt, Bill, Jr., and Steve. "Billy told me he had a hard time sleeping the first night, realizing how much Bill does depend on us," Carol says. "I think it was kind of hard on him. It really hit him. It was the same for Matt and Steve, that realization of what it's all about."

But watching their father deal with his lot with the same equanimity and grace he'd shown throughout his life helped the family accept the situation. "What I have learned from him since his diagnosis exceeds anything he taught me before," says Bill, Jr. "He has not given up hope and he refuses to let the disease stop him from living. He continues to stay active any way he can and he still plays an important role in my life. I still seek advice from him, and he's always happy to help me. Talking to him always brightens my day, and I cherish every moment I spend with him."

Here at the Center for BrainHealth, we deal with brave, intelligent, strong people every day. But the Tuels stand out, not only as a couple dealing with their own struggles, but because they are always ready to reach out and educate others on what Alzheimer's is, what it isn't, and how to make the best of life despite it.

Sometimes, as Bill's daughter, Kristin, points out, education is all that is necessary to change minds about the things that frighten us. "Before the diagnosis we knew something was wrong but we did not know what to do and it was hard to talk about it," she says. "Alzheimer's was a frightening word, a terrifying concept. Knowing, facing, and dissecting it has shifted that power. It is what it is, no greater than the sum of its parts, an organic process that may never be fully understood or ameliorated. It can rob families, but it doesn't have to."

Despite his rough road to retirement from work, the diagnosis of Alzheimer's has not caused Bill to retire from life. Instead, it has given him a new challenge to find ways to continue to give back. We all need a purpose, and Bill's spirit continues to inspire me. Bill's consistent queries about the status of this book underline its importance to him. To him, this book represents another opportunity to help people.

That is the kind of clear thinking and courage that keeps our clients—and their loved ones—looking to the future with hope instead of despair.

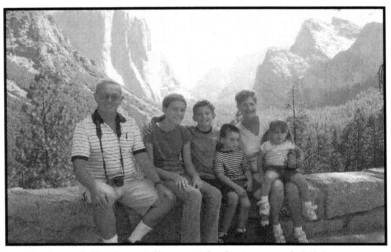

Jack and Shirley Kalling with their grandchildren at
Yosemite National Park.

*With his methodical, problem-solving mind,
Jack Kalling invents ways to work around Primary
Progressive Aphasia.*

Chapter 8
Engineering Hope

"If you don't have what you need, improvise!"
Jack Kalling

Jack Kalling lives by the Boy Scout motto, and everyone who knows him describes him as steady, reliable, dignified—and funny. An oil and gas engineer and avid car enthusiast, Jack's gift has always been his ability to solve any problem he puts his orderly mind to work on.

In a Stark Club meeting not long ago, I mentioned my favorite flavor of pie was rhubarb, although I had tasted it only once in my life.

The next meeting, Jack brought me a rhubarb pie he had baked himself. I was so touched—and impressed. Primary Progressive Aphasia (PPA) has interfered with Jack's ability to communicate verbally and it was taking some toll on his cognitive clarity, but his steel-trap engineer's mind could still follow a recipe. That pie was delicious!

I called Jack later that day to thank him again and tell him how good the pie was. Although he couldn't respond verbally, his wife, Shirley, told me he was beaming and giving her the thumbs-up as I spoke. A little while later I got an email from Jack. It included the recipe and said:

Hi Audette,

I hear pie good on phone!

Sincerely,

Jack

The members of the Stark Club never fail to amaze and surprise me.

A Scout is trustworthy, loyal, helpful, friendly, courteous, kind, obedient, cheerful, thrifty, brave, clean, and reverent. Before PPA robbed Jack of speech, he could rattle those words off at lightning speed—he learned them during his days as a Boy Scout in San Diego. And they weren't just words to him. "He has always lived by the Boy Scout code," Shirley says. Jack's mother describes her son as "calm, thoughtful, trustworthy, dependable—perfect and steady." And when Shirley first met Jack, he informed her he was perfect, adding with typical dry wit, "If you don't believe me, just ask me." Jack is one of the most persistent people you could ever hope to meet.

Jack's *Collection of Life Stories* book is full of adventures—camping and mountain climbing, scouting and flying—even a close encounter with a bear. He has also been a scout an educator and an engineer at Shell Oil.

And Jack is an innovator and a creative thinker in every way. His sister Linda Skoglund reminisces about a gift Jack gave her for Christmas when they were teenagers. "It was a work of art!" she exclaims. "Jack carefully cut and fashioned boxes and cylinders, wrapped them in tissue paper and decorated the face and body to look like a delightful little animal." (Inside the creative package was a new tennis racket.) Jack was "Uncle Jack" to the sons of close friend Ross and Nancy Radcliffe, and Uncle Jack used to thrill the boys, who were crazy for Teenage Mutant Ninja Turtles, by making green, turtle-shaped pancakes.

Engineers might have a reputation for being dry and colorless but Jack defies that stereotype in every way. However, if you were to meet Jack now, you would find him hard to read. He has limited facial expression these days and on first meeting you wouldn't get a sense of how fun he is. When words started failing Jack in 1999, he at first denied it and insisted Shirley's hearing was the problem.

"I was the only one who noticed it," Shirley recalls. "My girls didn't notice it, he didn't notice it. I was the only one. But I kept after him." Jack saw a doctor who recommended he get more rest, but that didn't work. "I would still correct him," Shirley says. "The girls would get mad at me. They thought I was being over-reactive."

Shirley, who is a special education teacher, continued to find cause for concern, yet the more she encouraged Jack to go to the doctor, the angrier he became. Shirley remembers telling Jack, "If something is really wrong, I will be the most understanding wife in the world, but if something is not wrong, something's got to give because this is not working."

By late 2001, even Jack realized something was wrong, and through a friend of his daughter was connected with a neurologist and specialists at the Center for BrainHealth. In 2002, when he was sixty-one, Jack was diagnosed with PPA.

"It was terribly frustrating and emotionally painful for probably two years," remembers Shirley. Jack was utterly resistant to the diagnosis—and angry. "He denied it, he said there is nothing wrong, I will get better, it's just a speech problem, it's just vitamins," Shirley says. And he blamed her for the diagnosis. "He said, 'If you had not talked to the doctors, I would not have this diagnosis. I was as understanding as I could be, but then my emotions got in the way, too. I got very frustrated."

Nevertheless, Jack immediately put his engineer's mind to understanding the disease and researching his options. "My engineer training looks for root causes," Jack has written about that time. He researched PPA on the Internet. "I learned about brain plasticity, which gave me hope," he wrote. "I tried fighting the disease by following the advice of doctors. I enrolled in speech therapy at a university clinic close to my house."

At speech therapy, says Shirley, "because he's so bright, knowledgeable, and cooperative and he worked so hard, I really think they thought that he could improve. They weren't sure about the diagnosis." And that, of course, fueled Jack's quest for a way out of the diagnosis.

"He wanted to do anything and everything he could," Shirley says. "I was told that all of our money would be gone by the time he died. I didn't care if we were totally broke because if there was something out there, then fine. And if that gave him hope, then that's fine. But I knew the reality."

When the couple discussed the diagnosis with us at the Center for BrainHealth, we suggested Jack come to a Stark Club meeting. Jack wasn't enthusiastic, but agreed to give it a try. After his first meeting, he came home doubtful. "He wasn't sure he needed the group," Shirley recalls. "He really enjoyed the meeting because Wayne Smith was in the group and he was an admiral and had PPA. But otherwise he said, 'I don't need this because there's nothing wrong with me.'"

My colleague, Stephanie, encouraged Jack to give the Stark Club three meetings before he made the decision about whether to stay. By the third visit, he was hooked—but less for the support he got than the support he felt he could provide to others. "He felt like the star pupil," Shirley says. "He felt like he could help the others and saw the group not as a place for him to get help, but a place for him to help the people who were helping the other people. He felt like he was kind of like an assistant leader and he took that role very seriously because that was what he used to do at Shell."

One of the tasks Jack undertook for himself and the other members of the Stark Club was reading technical books and articles about the brain and summarizing them. Eventually, though, the articles became so complex that Stark Club member Bill Crist pulled Jack aside and suggested that some of the articles were beyond some of their fellow club members' comprehension abilities.

So much of Jack's cognitive strengths remained for so long after his diagnosis that his boss at Shell Oil, for whom he had been doing consulting after his retirement in 1999, simply refused to let Jack resign. "His boss, Mike Jones, said, 'I know Jack and I know what he can do. I know not to give him any assignments where he has to talk or get up in front of the group, but his technical writing skills are still intact,'" Shirley recalls.

The semester we worked on the *Collection of Life Stories* with the Stark Club members, it was soon evident that Jack had his own ideas of how the book should be constructed. He had a long list of story ideas for his book. The stories were still alive in his mind, but because of PPA, his ability to tell them was diminished. The book was a great project for Jack and occupied him for years. In fact, he continues to add to the book, looking for pictures to go with the stories, investigating pertinent details, and scanning the pictures into the computer. But the stories have changed over the years. "You can see his (disease) progression in the book," comments Shirley. "The initial stories are more expansive, and as time has continued the stories are shorter and have incorrect grammar."

———

In many ways, Jack has simply refused to succumb to the diagnosis. He's not angry anymore, and he is aware that his speech is affected, but he does not acknowledge any other ways the disease is changing him. This is not an entirely bad thing for Jack because it keeps him going and engaged, but it is an ongoing challenge for Shirley, who has in a sense become an engineer herself, devising strategies and systems to help Jack without damaging his confidence and hope.

In addition to denying problems with his speech, Jack overestimates his declining cognitive abilities. His denial of his problems, coupled with his tendency to get obsessive when he has an idea, can be challenging. Although he has given up his car keys, he still insists on taking solo cycling treks. On one occasion, Jack broke a jar of spaghetti sauce and instead of waiting on Shirley to return to replace it, he decided to go to the store himself, which meant crossing a very busy four-lane street.

One result of the dementia is an inability to see reason or see another person's viewpoint, which can result in the person being inflexible. An example of his inflexibility happened as they were planning a family trip to Yosemite National Park, where Jack wanted to show his grandkids the spots he enjoyed camping as a boy. He also wanted to repeat a dangerous hike on Half Dome, a seventeen-mile hike that is grueling for people with all of their capabilities. Shirley knew trying to stop him once they were at Yosemite would be difficult. "I resigned myself. If something happens, it happens," she says. A bout of pneumonia interfered with his hiking plans, although he did accomplish his goal of sharing the park with his grandchildren. And Shirley was relieved to be spared the battle.

Shirley's proactive approach to the disease has avoided difficulty in another area—the Internet. Shirley discovered Jack had established email contact with a Cadillac dealership in an effort to find a 2006 Pontiac G-6 convertible. "It reminds him of the car he had when he first met me," Shirley says. She called the dealership to explain his dementia, and the dealership was incredibly kind, saying Jack could continue to write, but they would not sell him a car.

Shirley has developed her philosophy of dealing with the disease. "If he doesn't feel he's in control over his environment—and that's all he wants, control and independence—then we'll have behavior problems. I try to arrange the environment so Jack can have the perception he is in control, but I have to always be behind or beside and make sure I have back-up." For example, on a recent trip to Houston for a reunion of Shell associates, Jack had a folder containing all the information they needed, including hotel information Shirley gave him. But when they arrived in Houston, the hotel information was missing from the folder. They drove around for ninety minutes looking for the hotel before Shirley finally found the information in the back seat. "It will always be frustrating. It was my fault because I didn't make a second copy of the information."

Jack also wants control over the finances. He doesn't pay the bills, but insists on downloading the information to Quicken so he can work with it. At first, he frequently forgot their PIN and locked them out of their bank account. Shirley addressed this problem by going to the bank and getting a separate PIN for herself. When Jack locked himself out, he tried to figure out her PIN. "I have to hide the information so Jack won't lock me out," Shirley says.

But these necessary adaptations and unavoidable frustrations are only part of life with Jack. Though he can no longer drive his beloved vintage Studebaker, he still enjoys participating in meetings of the Studebaker Club. He and Shirley still love throwing parties for the Stark Club and for the San Diego State University alumni association, of which Jack is a member, which comes to Texas from time to time for football games. The Kallings put a great deal of thought into their parties.

Jack makes extensive lists and plans for every party, even if he doesn't always accomplish all he hopes. After a Stark Club cookout, he sent me a list of all the things he forgot to do, including:

I didn't wear Barbeque Hall of Flame apron.

I left the brain Jell-O in the fridge.

I didn't remind us to call Wayne and Molly.

I didn't give out the Panhandle marinade recipe.

Jack has always been a list-maker and a schedule-keeper, and Shirley has capitalized on this aptitude and created a system that works well for them. One of the first things she did after Jack was diagnosed was get a spiral notebook in which to combine their individual date books. Each day, they put a line down the center of the page and list Jack's activities for the day on one side and Shirley's on the other. Activities they will do together go in the center of the page, and Jack adds his television schedule on the bottom of the page. Jack's side of the page might include such chores as maintaining their swimming pool, taking out the trash, pulling weeds and planting flowers, although Shirley says that he is better at doing tasks she assigns him than at initiating chores himself—but, she adds with a laugh, "He makes his own coffee. I'm not allowed to make the coffee."

As Jack's disease progressed and Shirley became less comfortable about leaving him alone, she hired a man to spend several hours a week with Jack. Jack, of course, doesn't view this man as a hired companion but as a hired handyman who helps around the house with chores and maintenance. "Jack doesn't like not being able to do what he wants to do, so now one day a week, he can," Shirley says.

Shirley also quickly realized that Jack's ability to write things down long outlasted his ability to express himself verbally. From early on, when Shirley couldn't understand what he was trying to say, she would hand him a pencil and paper and ask him to write it down. Jack's computer skills also remained strong, and he frequently uses email to communicate. After Wayne and Molly Smith moved away, Jack kept them updated on Stark Club activities via emailed notes and photos.

Jack now carries notepads everywhere he goes to help him communicate, leaving behind drifts of paper with his comments, thoughts, questions. After our interview for this book, I was left with a small pile of yellow lined papers with Jack's contributions to our conversation. "Family support!!" reads one. "Shirley get traffic ticket today," was a sly poke at his wife, but all was smoothed over. "You love me," he affirmed on another slip of paper.

Shirley also discovered, as Jack's PPA progressed, that she needed to use short, emphatic sentences when talking to him, gently emphasizing content words. "For example, I might say, 'Jack I'm going to *lunch*. I'll be *back* at *one*. Be *ready*,'" she explains. "And I know when he's gotten it and I know when he hasn't. When all else fails, I use affection. I take his hand. I always try to make eye contact."

Shirley understands what Jack is trying to say even when nobody else can. "I know his interests," she says. "I realize that I know even more about him than I thought I did. I know more about his work than I thought I did. I figure out what he's saying through context. If someone else is having a conversation and he says something, I can pick out a word or a phrase and figure out how it applies to what we were talking about. There really is an advantage to having been married to him for forty-two years!"

Eventually, the Kallings got Jack a speech generating device (SGD), which creates electronic speech. He types words and sentences into the device, then hits a button to let the machine speak for him. The first sentences Jack programmed into his SGD were "I love you" for Shirley; their daughters, Danica and Marcy; their grandkids, Lorelle, Colin, Coleman, Morgan, and Drayton; and other family members. Jack took to the SGD so enthusiastically (that engineer's mind again—he loves a good gizmo) that Shirley wishes they had gotten it sooner.

The device allows Jack to participate more fully in the Stark Club meetings. Each week the Stark Club members have an assignment for the next meeting. Jack is able to program his answers into the machine prior to the meeting. He lets me know with a raised finger when he has programmed a comment in, then I give him a signal when it's a good time for him to hit the play button.

Jack has always been a problem solver and this trait has served him well. And in Jack's case, perhaps a little bit of denial is a good thing. He remains motivated to keep learning, keep experimenting, and keep finding ways to maintain his hope.

"Jack could have become discouraged and bitter, even given up," observes his sister, Linda. "But there is tenacity in his spirit that gives him strength to keep on going. No matter what he confronts—using his mechanical expertise in designing a project or dealing with the unexplainable encumbrances of life—Jack perseveres with sustained patience and determination."

I asked Jack and Shirley what advice they had for couples just embarking on the journey they have been forced to take. Shirley groped to respond. "I don't have a lot of time to think about what I do or what I should be doing because I'm just living it," she says. "This may not be what we want and the outcome might not be what we want. We thought we'd spend the next thirty years traveling and doing fun things. But everything's going to be all right. We're going to be all right. Instead of trying to fight the inevitable, let's make it a friend and we can live with it. Let's make it a part of who we are, let's laugh about it. Our faith gets us through these tough times."

"Positive!" Jack wrote on a piece of yellow paper, placing it in front of me emphatically.

Once again, I can only be impressed.

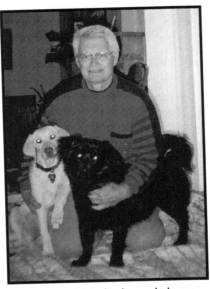

Stan and his beloved dogs.

Stan Fedyniak found time for pleasant new pursuits when Lewy body disease forced him to slow his pace.

Chapter 9
Seize the Day

*"Sometimes you just have to laugh at yourself—
relax!" Stan Fedyniak*

*In his long career in retail, Stan Fedyniak was known as
the guy who could sell shoes to a man with no feet. At home,
he has always been the go-to guy for household projects and
repairs. A former Marine (Semper Fi), Stan is practical and
reliable—a quiet guy with a deep well of strength.*

Stan is the thinker; his wife Dawn is the talker.
Sometimes, though, as Dawn chatters away—and Stan
talks even less since he was diagnosed with Lewy Body
disease—expressions pass across Stan's face that leave no
mistake what he's thinking.

When Dawn once told me, "These days, whatever I say
goes," Stan's sly and indulgent smile made Dawn laugh,
suggesting a long-standing joke in their marriage. And
when she said, "I talk incessantly and he tunes me out,"
Stan chuckled and she joined him. And once, when Dawn

and Stan were seeing a physical therapist who suggested a wheelchair for Stan, Dawn thought it was a good idea, but Stan did not. "Oh boy, did I get the look!" Dawn recalls. No, Stan did not want a wheelchair, and he let Dawn know with just a pointed glance.

Communication between couples is never limited to just words, and intimacy in a marriage is not entirely contingent on conversation. In some ways, since Stan's diagnosis, the Fedyniaks have discovered new facets to their marriage. For the first time since they met and married, Dawn and Stan have something they never had before: time.

———

Stan and Dawn both have worked full-time through most of their marriage. Stan was always a very hard worker in his retail career with such companies as Knapp Shoes, Montgomery Ward, Dollar General, and others. Retail is often a six-day-a-week job, and as a manager, Stan often had to travel. The family rarely took vacations. On Sundays, when Stan was home, chores, honey-dos and their daughter, Tanya, kept Stan and Dawn busy and focused on everything but each other.

As is common when dementia strikes at a young age, it was problems at work that first got Stan and Dawn's attention. Stan started having trouble holding jobs. "He couldn't keep them, or he knew he couldn't do them, and so he would say, 'I'm just going to move on to something else,'" Dawn recalls. He went through a half dozen jobs, lasting only a couple of years at each.

"I thought, 'Geez, retail has really changed,'" Dawn says. "It was always difficult, but the demands they put on him these days...what's the deal? But I always excused it, thinking it was just retail. But then he'd make some little remark about how he got lost or something. I kept saying to him, 'You're tired. When you get that tired you can't function.' I'd say, 'Sleep the weekend away.' And he'd sleep and sleep and sleep, but it was never enough sleep."

In 2003, when he was sixty, Stan was demoted from his store manager position to a minimum wage job on the sales floor. He quit that job, but Dawn was surprised when he put no effort into finding another job. "I watched him sleep and roam around the house, lost and defeated," she recalls.

It was at that time that she remembered a public television program she had seen that talked about Alzheimer's and the Center for BrainHealth and she decided it was time to face a lurking fear.

Through testing here, Stan was diagnosed with Alzheimer's and within one year he was re-diagnosed with Lewy Body disease, the second most common form of dementia. In addition to the memory problems associated with Alzheimer's disease, individuals with Lewy Body disease can exhibit Parkinson's-like symptoms.

I am pleased to hear how warmly Dawn recalls the sensitivity of the round table meeting when the diagnosis was explained to the couple. "It was amazing how it was handled," she remembers. "Rather than say he couldn't work anymore, they said 'we'—meaning everyone involved—'would have to think of other ways you could bring income into the house, such as VA and Social Security.' And when they talked about not driving anymore, they said, 'Remember how you would drive and get lost and how anxious and scared you were? We don't want that to happen anymore.'"

Of course, Stan understood exactly how his life was changing, and Dawn saw tears in his eyes. Then their daughter, Tanya, who was twenty-seven at the time, said, "Dad, you've worked so hard for so long, why don't you think of retiring? Now is the time to start doing all those things you like but never had time for."

Those were like magic words, Dawn recalls, and they calmed Stan right down.

To some extent, the diagnosis was a relief because it explained everything that had been happening. "And then we thought, OK, this is our life, now we have to go forward with it," Dawn says.

And they did.

———

Stan did retire, although Dawn kept working as an executive legal assistant, and the couple's life took on a more leisurely pace. "It was nice to have him home," Dawn says.

Stan was comfortable being alone all day while Dawn was working. He still was able to do some home repairs and for his first project as a homebody, he decided to make improvements to their backyard. "I knew what I wanted to do," our man of few words says—and he was not thinking in terms of puttering, but major landscaping. He surprised Dawn when he took their wheelbarrow half a mile down the street to a construction site and hauled home enormous boulders for his project. Dawn would come home from work and find that he'd moved monumental stones into their yard. "I'd ask him, 'How did you get that home?'" Dawn marvels. "And he said, 'I just took special steps and I took breaks.' It was amazing. And it went on for weeks."

Sometimes Dawn—the eternal cheerleader who loved seeing Stan engaged in his project—would drive him around to other building sites to find more boulders, which they loaded into the trunk or back seat of the car. He rearranged the landscaping ties and planted the flowers and foliage Dawn bought for him. "He created an even more beautiful backyard," Dawn says with pride.

Although Stan struggles with other repairs and projects, Dawn makes a concerted effort to keep him engaged in the household so he knows he is still important. For example, "one beautiful Saturday morning I asked Stan if he would replace the ripped vacuum belt for me," she says. "He had been sitting idle and lost, so I thought I'd give him an assignment. Since I already knew how to replace the belt, I thought I'd give him something to work on that used to be easy for him. We carried the vacuum outside and placed it on the patio table. I had the tools handy. I left him alone with the job. Stan looked at the vacuum for at least ten minutes before he decided to begin work on it. I then asked if I could watch, so I could learn how to do it. He said OK. I watched as he began the correct procedure for the repair—although it did take a long time. He was always very careful with any repairs. He explained the procedure and said to always make sure that when making repairs, the vacuum is not plugged in. In his own way, he was telling me he was still being careful. He did all the right things." Dawn was proud of Stan, even though when she thanked him again ten minutes later, he didn't remember doing the job.

———

The Fedyniaks joined the Stark Club soon after Stan's diagnosis and rely on it for support and camaraderie.

Stan took to the group right away. "It was a place to talk to people," he says. "The thoughts come out and I can feel the friendship there." Even though Stan is quiet and shy, he is clearly engaged in the discussions even if he doesn't always contribute. He is also well educated and when he does speak, he shares his thoughts passionately and eloquently.

And Dawn, despite her full-time job, always takes time out of her work week to come to the Stark Club with Stan. She treasures her time visiting with the other caregivers. Dawn sorely misses the interaction during stretches when Stan is too ill to attend, or when we go on hiatus, and she makes an effort to stay in touch with other members via email or telephone during those times.

Aside from the Stark Club, the Fedyniaks find that they are perfectly content spending most of their time in the company of each other and their dogs. The first dog Stan and Dawn took in was actually Tanya's. She let her Sasha stay with Stan, after he received his dementia diagnosis, for several months to keep him company, and when she tried to bring her back home, Stan put on a sad face. Tanya went shopping for a dog for her Dad, without telling her Mom until after the fact. Tanya was ready to take her dog back. Dawn wasn't fond of dogs at that point (she soon changed), but told Tanya, "That's a beautiful thing to do." Tanya never got her Sasha back. Stan still has both of them! "We often joke about how Tanya's Sasha came to spend the weekend with Papa, and stayed three years," Dawn says.

Stan was worried that if he came up with a new name for his new dog he wouldn't be able to remember it, so with Tanya's permission, he named his new best friend Sasha II. A while later, Tanya added dog number three, Sam, to the family, who also spends a lot of time with Stan.

"I can't imagine life without them," Dawn says. "The dogs are Stan's life. They are the ones that stay with him, and he depends on them. If they could administer medical help, they would. He's never alone. He goes to bed, they're with him. He gets up, they're with him. If they move ahead of him, they turn around to make sure he's still there." (Dawn admits with a laugh that she has had to move into another bedroom since there is no longer room for her in their queen-size bed.)

And Stan—who was never one to go out with the guys or juggle a complex social life—likes the company of canines and the quiet life perfectly well. Though he's home alone all day, he doesn't complain of loneliness. "I don't get bored, I don't cry," he says. "I just have fun with the pups, I read the paper, I sleep."

Tanya also is an important part of her dad's life. She is and always has been a daddy's girl. She calls her dad every morning and again later in the day. And Dawn and Stan have developed their own daily rituals. "We seem to have developed a routine when I come home from work every day," Dawn says. "We gather on the patio with the Sashas. Stan always begins with, 'How was your day?'" I'll tell him, even though he doesn't always follow it. Then, we move on to the Sashas—how much he loves them and what great company they are. We talk about nature—the birds that come to visit, and I question him about why birds do certain things. Stan loves nature, and I try to make sure he knows that whatever he says or contributes is very important."

And Stan knows that. "That's why I talk to you," he says. "I've got two pups to talk to, but I talk to you!"

Dawn beams at the words. "I like that," she says. "I like to hear his voice. The life we have is pretty much each other. And anything material doesn't matter, never did matter."

And interestingly, Dawn is finding that with their newfound leisure time together, the new challenges of communicating with Stan, and the changes in Stan's capabilities and interests, their relationship is actually growing in ways she never expected. Because Stan was away from home so much when he was still working, she became accustomed to doing things her own way and was even a little hardheaded about it. "He would say, 'Whatever, do what you want,' but I started to realize that I didn't really let him express himself. He dealt me the cards and I had to become controlling. He went to his job and I did everything else."

But now, Dawn is more anxious to solicit his input on things. "I try to ask him questions, especially if I have to make a decision. He used to be able to give some really good pointers, and sometimes he still can. It's always a surprise every day. You never know. I know there's still fire in the furnace there. I can tell it by his facial expressions."

And, she says, she's become more easygoing in general because she's more focused on appreciating what is rather than what she wishes would be. "I'm actually listening to what people are trying to say, and I try and make positive comments rather than a criticism," she says. Even when Stan says something that is—shall we say—less than diplomatic, Dawn finds it easier to laugh off than she once might have. "Like he might say, 'Looks like you've put on weight,' and I'll say, 'I know, doesn't it look good?' rather than make a scene, which doesn't change anything. Day to day, minute to minute—that's how I live, and as long as he can talk to me, I'm happy."

Stan also seems more easygoing—sometimes even sillier—than he used to be. Once at a Stark Club party to which he'd neglected to bring a bathing suit, he so wanted to join a free-form volleyball game in the swimming pool that he finally just jumped in fully clothed, except for his shoes. Dawn was surprised—Stan could be impulsive in the past, but not often. But she could only laugh and love it—what are wet clothes when everyone was having such fun? "I do stupid things like that," Stan says with a grin. "I'm not that inhibited."

"We laugh a lot," Dawn says. "If Stan had not continued with his normal easygoing manner, I don't think we would be laughing so much."

And after the laughter, the couple often takes the time to express their love. "To this day Stan understands, without my saying anything," Dawn says. "He feels the pressure I'm under. He says things like, 'You work so hard to take care of me and everything else. No wonder you are tired and have no time for yourself.'" While comments like this don't change anything, technically, they are nourishment for Dawn's soul and help her keep going.

Despite the fear that accompanies a dementia diagnosis, Dawn and Stan and Tanya, too, have discovered new depths to their relationships with each other. And the dogs, of course.

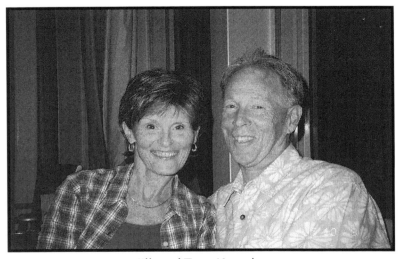

Jill and Tom Keppler

Quiet, Tom Keppler, didn't forsake the physical activities he loved after a diagnosis of Alzheimer's disease.

Chapter 10
Staying the Course

"The commitment to do something is good."
Tom Keppler

Tom Keppler's Collection of Life Stories *book contains a photograph of his first bicycle. Also his second bicycle. And it includes descriptions of races he's been in and cycling trips he's taken, including one from California to Florida. Tom has ridden in eight national parks—startling bears and cougars along the way—and he even commuted by bicycle to work for awhile, riding a total of twenty-five miles a day. An accountant by trade, Tom is an athlete at heart.*

You don't become a different person after you get a diagnosis of Alzheimer's disease. In many ways, the aspects of what define a person throughout life may actually become more apparent after a diagnosis, when other aspects of a person's life fall away.

Family and friends define Tom by his love for family and adventure, and these loves remain strong three years after his diagnosis and ten years after he started showing signs of Alzheimer's. While Alzheimer's does initiate change, the diagnosis doesn't have to take over completely for people who learn how to modify their lives to accommodate the disease. Tom and his wife, Jill, are a team, navigating the ever-changing course of Alzheimer's by anchoring themselves to the people and activities they love.

Jill, who teaches mentally challenged and autistic children, and Tom both had been married once before when they met at work. Tom was too shy to approach Jill directly, so one of his work buddies broke Tom's pencils repeatedly, forcing Tom to visit the pencil sharpener by Jill's desk until finally he got up the nerve to ask her out. Tom needed a little nudge to get things started, but Jill's love for the outdoors quickly clinched the romance.

"When Tom and I had our first date, he said, 'I can't believe it...you love the outdoors?'" Jill remembers. "'You really like to camp and canoe?'"

"I had trouble meeting girls who liked camping and stuff," Tom says.

Jill even took up cycling for her handsome new boyfriend. "It was part of our courtship," she says. "He bought me my first official bicycle." The couple went for long rides together, "I didn't have the confidence, but he said, 'Oh yes, you can do it,'" Jill says. "And he got our friends involved. He was always the one who'd go up the hill and then come down to check on everybody."

In 1977, the couple married, blending their families—Jill's daughter, Ashley (two years old at the time), and Tom's three children, Jim (age nine), Amy (age eight), and Cara (age six)—and embarking on a loving, faith-filled, and active life together. In 1981, they had another child, John.

———

Life rolled along pleasantly for decades until Tom started having cognitive difficulties—long before his diagnosis. He had trouble remembering their home alarm code and trouble keeping things straight and organized at his job as an accountant for General Motors. But Jill, as so often happens when Alzheimer's strikes young, didn't think the problems were anything to get worked up about.

"He was always my financial man," Jill says. "He did a lot of computer work, he had these detailed spreadsheets. I remember he kept saying 'Jill, you need to learn this stuff, you need to learn this stuff.' I could see some slippage. He would come home from work and say, 'Something's just not clicking.' Little things accumulated, but I kind of put it on the back burner."

Jill came up with every possible explanation for the creeping problems. She thought it might be stress, depression, or boredom. "He kept saying he was bored on his job," she recalls. For nearly six years, she didn't suspect the real cause. "I never thought it was neurological," she says, shaking her head.

But the problems eventually took a toll on Tom's physical activities and that's when Jill began taking note. When he painted their house, it took him two weeks just to paint the trim. After taking an early retirement buyout from a job with GM, he started interviewing for other jobs, including one to drive Leaseway trucks. "He came home and said, 'I had difficulty backing the truck up,'" Jill recalls. "It wasn't a big semi. It was a small one. This was a man who used to drive a motor home."

Tom decided to build a deck for their home. "I remember coming home after work, and saying, 'You only installed two planks today!'" Jill says. "I remember him juggling a drill back and forth between his left and right hands. Tom is a lefty. He couldn't decide which hand to use. He's always been very dexterous. Always. When things like that started popping up, that was really a red flag."

The evidence continued adding up in the sort of frightening litany familiar to anyone who has witnessed the onset of dementia. The first person to suggest the possibility of Alzheimer's disease was the Kepplers' daughter, Cara, a nurse. In April 2002, after noticing that her father became confused while playing a familiar game, she had her dad draw the face of a clock, a standard task in a neurological exam. Tom drew an oval clock with all the numbers on the left side.

Soon after, Tom and Jill saw a neurologist and Alzheimer's expert at Illinois University Medical Center (the couple lived in Indiana at the time). Tom underwent six stressful hours of testing. "I remember the depressed look on Tom's face when he finished," Jill says. "He said, 'I felt like an idiot! I don't want to go through that ever again!'"

Even after all that testing, the doctor suggested that Tom's problems might be Alzheimer's, but that he wasn't ready to rule out depression yet. He prescribed antidepressants for Tom, pointing out that if depression was the problem, they would see improvement in a few months. Tom protested that he was not depressed. "How could I be?" he said. "I have a wonderful wife and five wonderful children!"

Tom was right—depression wasn't the problem. In January of 2003, when Tom was sixty years old, the neurologist diagnosed him with Alzheimer's disease.

———

After Tom's diagnosis, in July 2003, the Kepplers moved to Texas from Indiana to escape the cold winters, which kept Tom indoors, and to be closer to their daughter, Ashley. They chose a gated community that felt safe and comfortable to Jill, who was concerned about leaving Tom home alone during the day.

"I felt instantly pretty secure about him living here. It's gated, and there are a lot of people home during the day because they're retired," she says. The community also has a clubhouse with a fitness center that Tom could easily get to, so he could maintain the exercise program that is so integral to who he is.

At first, Tom was reluctant to go out into the neighborhood on his own. "I tried teaching him ways he could drive in the neighborhood, but he couldn't remember how to get home," says Jill. "I remember thinking: I've made a mistake moving him from familiar territory. Thank God his love for exercise and the outdoors motivated him to learn his way around the neighborhood."

Jill sometimes worried that while she was at work Tom would hop on his bike and take off, but so far that hasn't happened "that I know of," she says. He did start walking to and from the clubhouse fitness center, keeping to walking paths and finding his way there and back without mishap.

———

Tom is not much quieter today than he was before his diagnosis, and his eyes still twinkle as always. But today, his silence isn't just introversion.

"It's like he's deep in thought all the time," says Jill. "He's always been like that, but in the past when he was thinking about something, eventually he would share with me what was on his mind. But now it's like he's in his own little world."

Still, that world did not need to be an isolated place and Tom reaches out in his own ways. The Kepplers, like all our Stark Club members, pay attention to new research and retain hope for themselves and for others afflicted with the disease. To that end, shortly after his diagnosis, Tom entered a four-month clinical trial for a new drug. "If I can help with the possibility of this being a cure for other people, I want to do it," he says.

Tom and Jill came to the Stark Club shortly after their move to Dallas. They were introduced to the club by Bill and Carol Tuel after the two couples met at a support group near their home. They have since forged a strong friendship.

"We felt very isolated when Tom started having problems," Jill says. "I don't think our friends knew what to do, especially after we got the diagnosis. I remember how lonely I was. I wanted a friend or a group that I could talk to. The Stark Club has been such a blessing. It's our core social group. It seems like we're doing something every weekend with either the Tuels or someone from the Stark Club."

Just as Tom introduced Jill to biking early in their courtship, the Kepplers wanted to pass their love of the outdoors to their new friends, so Jill organized a float trip down the Comal River for the Stark Club. This was a new activity for most of the couples, but they embraced the idea with enthusiasm. Even though the trip had to be cancelled due to heavy rains, the process of planning and the anticipation of adventure provided an incredible bonding experience for the group. The focus was on considering the possibilities.

Jill wanted Tom to continue cycling without her, but she was concerned about him getting lost. Seeking to maintain his independence and address her concern of leaving Tom at home alone while she was at work, Jill hired a companion who was willing to double as a trainer. On the first day the trainer showed up, he borrowed one of Tom's bikes. "Tom was going to show him around the neighborhood. I didn't count on Tom's peak physical condition being a problem," Jill recalls. "He got halfway down to the clubhouse, turned around, and the guy wasn't there."

Tom backtracked and found the trainer. "I thought he was going to die," Tom says, practically doubled over with laughter. "He had a cold or something. He was off his bike, huffing and puffing. We decided to go for a car ride instead." Jill and Tom decided to abandon the plan, but not cycling.

"We still take short rides weekly, a loop around the neighborhood that takes about forty-five minutes," Jill says. "And we've done some longer rides. We did one that was about twenty miles round trip. The heat bothers Tom, so we ride early in the morning."

In addition to cycling, Tom still works out daily, walking to the community health club to lift weights and to the pool to swim. "He's still lifting 290 pounds," Jill says. "He has no problems at the gym. They have a circuit. He does just fine there. He will stay on a spot for half an hour. He'll take his time, but that's always been his personality."

For as long as it was still enjoyable to Tom, he and Jill continued camping, but she remembers their last attempt at camping. "We took a hike, had a nice meal, then went to bed at about ten. Every hour after that, Tom was up going to the bathroom. It seemed all night long I was hearing zip, zip, zip of the tent flap. At 4 a.m., he said, 'Are we going home now? I'm ready to go home.'"

In the pitch dark, Tom struggled with stuffing the sleeping bags back into their cases and was unable to hold the flashlight steady for Jill to disassemble the tent. "The flashlight beam was high in the trees," Jill says. "I finally had to hold it in my mouth. That was a sad day because Tom and I loved camping."

Although Tom's level of participation in his long-loved activities has changed, he continues to enjoy talking about them in Stark Club meetings. One aspect of our meetings is spotlighting different group members and providing them the opportunity to discuss a topic of interest. For weeks before Tom's turn in the spotlight at the Stark Club, he updated me on the progress of a collage Jill was working on containing pictures and data on all his bike trips. He eagerly anticipated the day when he could share the information with the Stark Club.

These days, Tom gets his fix for adventure by reading, which he does voraciously. Books like *Into Thin Air,* John Krakauer's account of an ill-fated Mount Everest climb; *Blue Highways* by William Least Heat-Moon, about a trip on America's back roads; and *Dove* by Robin L. Graham, about an around-the-world sailing trip, help Tom keep in touch with his adventuresome side, and he is happy to read them over and over. Inspired by his love for adventure, the Stark Club at one point elected to read and discuss *Walk Across America* by Peter Jenkins.

Jill, too, has found the written word helpful. In her case, journaling has provided an outlet for her feelings and helps her keep in touch with where she's been on the journey with Alzheimer's. "I like reading back on feelings, on happy times, on general wisdom. And the Lord gave me words of wisdom and said, 'You're supposed to write a book,'" Jill says.

Faith, a powerful form of support for Jill and Tom throughout their lives, continues to provide comfort and strength. The couple prays together every morning. "If he has to stay home a little bit by himself, we always say a little prayer about that." The couple also attends Episcopalian services on Saturday nights. "The service is a little bit smaller and he likes that better," Jill says. "To this day, he still takes communion. He knows the proper way of walking up, though I go in front of him. There are ritual prayers and he still knows them without even reading them. This is all in his long-term memory. He's done quite well, even moving here and going to this new church."

Close family ties also keep the couple strong. When their daughter, Ashley, gave birth to twins in 2005, Tom was elated.

"The day that they were born we were at the hospital," Jill says. "Tom had tears in his eyes and said, 'Jill, this is going to put five years on my life.'" Tom now spends three days a week at Ashley's house while Jill is at work.

"Seeing him with Braeden and Payton reminds me of how my dad used to be," Ashley says. "He will sit and make silly faces at them and it feels good to see him happy." Ashley and her sisters, Cara and Amy, have tender memories of their dad from childhood. The three remember their dad letting them barber him and paint on his back with watercolors. They remember him giving them horsey rides. "My friends always loved to come over because none of their dads let us do these silly things. He has always been a kid at heart," Ashley says.

"I thought that in a lot of ways he was the complete package," says son Jim. "He's intelligent, handsome, athletic, sensitive, caring, strong. For the better part of my life, I thought my dad was invincible."

The Kepplers agree that despite his losses, Tom retains his finest qualities. "Dad's mind may be changing, but his soul is still the same," Amy says. "He's still someone to look up to and respect."

Meanwhile, Jill's long experience as a special education teacher has helped her. For example, she has figured out how to ease Tom's struggles with sequential tasks that are difficult for him.

Tom seems to do well with ritualistic activities, such as those at church. He takes the same route to the fitness center every times he goes, walks the dog along the same paths, and he still fixes his own breakfast of oatmeal, which he has eaten every morning for as long as Jill can remember.

Jill also has learned not to pressure Tom when she sees him getting frustrated. "Sometimes I don't think he knows that he's frustrated," she says. "Generally I just back off. Sometimes when I try to explain what's going on it just makes matters worse. It's a no-win situation."

Tom's quiet nature can be heartbreaking for Jill because he cannot express his feelings in words. Although he never has been voluble, she says, she could usually draw out his worries when she had to. Today, she says, "I can tell when he gets real upset, he'll go onto the patio and put his head on the table."

But even without words, the couple keeps the connection strong. Sometimes they just sit together on the sofa and hold each other. In the evenings, they walk the dog together or watch the sunset.

Jill says the disease's glacial pace is a blessing because it helps her adjust to one small change at a time. "It's like a hike," she says. "At some point, you hit the summit. We feel like in our marriage, we've hit the summit. We've had a good life and now we're on the downhill part of it. You have those level parts where you're stable, and you have these little drops. But God has been with us and even in those drops, I've always felt secure. You can't fear this disease. If you do, it will take all the joy out of life."

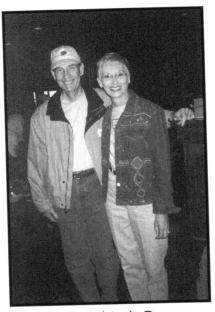

Delbert and Judy Duncan

Love of family defined Delbert Duncan and family made sure he was never left alone with his Alzheimer's disease.

Chapter 11
A Journey of Love

"I'm stuck on the family—that's what's important to me." Delbert Duncan

Steady, loving, and hard working, Delbert Duncan got his first job as a teenager to help with family expenses, spent forty-two years climbing the corporate ladder as a valued employee at Minyard Food Stores, and is a devoted husband and father. Delbert draws joy and energy from helping people, and his family especially has rallied around him to return that love.

Delbert and his wife, Judy, had no option but to discover together how to face Alzheimer's. But the couple was not alone on the journey. Instead of taking a back seat because they had never gone this way before, their family members rallied with compassionate involvement.

Working together, the entire extended family found ways to keep Delbert involved in his favorite activities, finding new ones in the process. This means that even as Delbert faces some losses, the Duncans make new discoveries about each other during this walk with Alzheimer's, which Judy views as a journey of love. When she wonders where to go next, she says, "We go wherever Delbert's fading memories take us—always thankful for the journey."

Delbert has always been a steady guy. His first job, at the age of fifteen, was sacking groceries at a local Minyard, a Dallas/Fort Worth area supermarket, and when he retired forty-two years later, he was still with the same company, although he had risen considerably in the ranks to senior vice president—administration.

Delbert could have been a very different kind of man with a different attitude towards work and family, considering his childhood. His family did not have a lot of money, his mother had a volatile personality. "My sisters left home as soon as they could," Delbert wrote in his *Collection of Life Stories* book. "My brother, Tom, kept me alive. I tried to help my mother, but I couldn't do anything about it. So I decided, I have to be me and I'm going to keep on going."

Delbert went to a rough high school in Dallas, where gangs reigned and the police were regular visitors (he often compared it to the movie *Blackboard Jungle*). And still, he kept going, holding two jobs as a teenager to help with family finances, putting himself through college, and making himself an indispensable employee at Minyard.

But it wasn't just Delbert's work ethic that helped him get ahead. Delbert's employers and the people who worked under him adored him because he was sensitive, caring, and interested in the people around him. As Delbert puts it, "I just like people."

In a way, Minyard was even responsible for Delbert meeting the love of his life, Judy. It all started as a joke. Delbert, who has a sly sense of humor that he shows only occasionally, told his secretary that he would fire her if she didn't find him a date. Delbert was teasing, but the young woman was gullible enough to tell Judy, who lived in the same apartment complex as she, that her job was at stake. So Judy helped her friend out and went out with Delbert. "We hit it off immediately," Judy says, and she didn't mind that Delbert already had two children from his first marriage. "I remember how much fun we had all going out on a date together," Judy recalls. The couple dated for three years and then married.

When Judy married Delbert, she added his two daughters, Melissa and Amy, to her family. When Delbert married Judy, he added her parents and sisters to his. And the combination has created a supportive, loving family that we all can learn from.

Delbert was still working and loving his job when the first symptoms of Alzheimer's started to show. His was, in a way, an unspectacular slip into the disease—memory problems, a tendency to seem a little bit "out there" as Judy describes it. "We'd talk about something and shortly later I'd bring it up again and it was new to him," she recalls. "That's what I noticed first."

Delbert was also having trouble contributing to meetings at work. "Probably it was more apparent to the people who worked for him, although it was never discussed with me," Judy says. "People were working around him. Maybe he didn't know that that was going on." Judy did notice problems with his memory and comprehension, but as I hear so often, she tried to tell herself that it would pass, that there were simple and fixable explanations. "I wanted to believe it was stress-related from work."

However, because Delbert's mother, brother, and one of his sisters all had Alzheimer's disease, Judy knew in the back of her mind and deep in her heart that the problems could be pointing to something more serious. At Judy's insistence, Delbert finally mentioned her concerns with his memory to their internist. After a series of interviews and tests with other doctors and neurologists, and about a year and a half after the Duncans first started noticing symptoms, Delbert was diagnosed with Alzheimer's. He was fifty-nine years old.

———

Needless to say, retiring in his fifties was not in Delbert's original life plan. In many ways, he was as dedicated to his job as he is to his family.

"My favorite thing about Minyard's is the individuals at the office," he wrote in his *Collection of Life Stories* book. "I made very close relationships and have some very good friends there. They've done a lot of things for me, and they are absolutely wonderful. I fell into it with all the good people. Minyard's is a very honest, close, family-owned company, and no one ever wants to retire; they all just get white hair!"

But also in Delbert's *Collection of Life Stories* book, one phrase crops up again and again, "I just keep going." And so, although he had to retire from Minyard after his diagnosis, he did just keep going. And, as he told Judy when we started talking about writing this book, "My diagnosis was not the end…but another chapter in my life—one that I hope can help others."

As Delbert wants to help others, so do others want to help him. Judy's family, who all live near the couple, rallied around as soon as the diagnosis was established. Their goals were not only to make sure that Delbert continued to have an active, engaged life, but also to make sure that Judy was supported and was able to continue doing the things outside the home that were important to her.

"We know that in many cases of an Alzheimer's diagnosis some family members pull away. Our family has always been extremely close and we all knew this would be when we would find out what *family* really means," says Judy's oldest sister, Cathey. She came up with the idea of getting a calendar together for the family and scheduling each member to spend time with Delbert in order to allow Judy to keep up with things that she enjoyed, such as volunteering at a hospital, which she has done for more than a decade. "Delbert likes me to do that and it's important to me," Judy says. "My family knew that and stepped up to help make sure I could continue."

The family has outings such as bowling, game, and movie night. Cathey and her husband, Ron, live across the street from Judy and Delbert and the two families frequently drop in to visit each other's homes. "Delbert has enjoyed being able to come to our home any time of the day or night," Cathey says. "We have many of our meals together. We laugh and have a great time."

Delbert's daughters and nieces find ways to continue spending time with him, such as taking him out to eat and shopping. They often helped him find the perfect gifts to give Judy for special occasions and holidays. And particularly touching is that when Cathey took Delbert along on errands, she would help him pick out special future birthday, anniversary, and Valentine's Day cards, which he would sign. Even after Delbert's impairment progressed to the point where he could no longer sign cards, Judy continues receiving these cards, signed in his own hand. "This has meant a great deal to me," she says.

Delbert's son-in-law, Scott, who also works for Minyard, would take Delbert to company functions so he could visit with friends and former coworkers. He also took Delbert fishing on a nearby lake.

Even little Ethan, the Duncans' youngest grandchild, who was born six years after Delbert was diagnosed, knows exactly who Grandad is because the family makes sure the two spend time together. And Delbert is, of course, a typically doting grandfather.

One of the most delightful ideas the family hatched was Judy's sister Connie's "Tuesdays with Delbert." Every Tuesday, until the progression of the disease made the work too stressful for Delbert, Connie and Delbert spent every Tuesday together doing good in their community.

"'Tuesdays with Delbert' was born out of the fact that I wanted to help him feel he still had a job in this world," Connie explains. "Delbert loves getting out and being around people. He had poured his life into his work at Minyard Foods and now he was lost without that. 'Tuesdays with Delbert' fell into place, giving him some freedom back. We would deliver Meals on Wheels to about fifteen or twenty shut-ins and help out at a food pantry. Delbert would greet each person with a smile and, 'How are you today?' No one ever knew his personal struggles."

Delbert never forgot his modest roots and got tremendous satisfaction out of reaching out to people who needed a helping hand, so delivering Meals on Wheels was ideal work for him, even though his tender heart was sometimes troubled by the things he saw. "I feel good when I do this," he wrote in his *Collection of Life Stories* book. "Some of the people we visit are farmers or former farmers. A lot of them live alone. We're not supposed to stop very long at each house, but we bend the rules. You just have to. We say hello and talk for a while. Sometimes you see things you wish were not there. We watch to see if people are eating their food. I think we help wherever we go. At Christmas time we wear Santa hats. It makes everybody smile."

Connie and Delbert also volunteered together at the Sharing Life Outreach Center, which provides food and clothing to people in need. "It's all they have," Delbert wrote. "We've got it and they don't. I don't like that. My family was poor for a long time when I was growing up. Now I like to see people make it."

What strikes me as particularly special about "Tuesdays with Delbert" is that not only did it get Delbert out with people—which has always been so important to him—but it also allowed him to continue doing the kind of outreach that was significant to him before his diagnosis. When he helped Minyard launch Carnival food stores, which target Hispanic consumers, Delbert felt good about providing a supermarket that made them feel at home. At the Sharing Life Center, many of the people who come for assistance are Hispanic. "I continue to serve the Hispanic community," Delbert wrote.

The Duncans also loved traveling before Delbert's diagnosis, partially motivated by his determination to see all fifty states. After his diagnosis they continued traveling. "I just stick close to his side," Judy says. They took a family cruise, all sixteen family members, including grandchildren, and Delbert and Judy often travel with Judy's parents. "They're in their early eighties and in great health. They're great companions and it's good to have them with us," Judy says.

———

Judy learned about the Stark Club through a support group for individuals with young-age-onset Alzheimer's. "I honestly don't know what people do if they don't have something this wonderful to be a part of," Judy says. "The Stark Club kept Delbert more outgoing. He can be very quiet, but he gets around people and he's energized. He's different around the Stark Club—more verbal and even acting goofy sometimes. I never know what he's going to say. He thrives on all that energy and it's good for him."

Combining their love of travel with the support they found at the Stark Club, the Duncans took a cruise with fellow Stark Club members the Kepplers and Tuels, knowing how helpful it is to be around other people who understand the challenges of dementia. "To be with first-time cruisers was such fun!" Judy says. "I'll admit the cruise was challenging, but knowing that it could very well be *our* last one, I was determined to make this week together as special as all the other cruises we had taken—Delbert's enjoyment in the moment and memories for *me* to hold on to long after."

The club has become an extension of family support. Though this wasn't why the club was started, it is an incredible dividend. And Judy is great at helping Delbert participate in Stark Club activities. She always makes sure to know what is happening in meetings so she can provide Delbert with information or contributions that will help him participate—like the time we were talking about the 1970s and she made sure Delbert brought in a photo of himself looking groovy in his 1970s leather jacket.

Judy also has benefited from the insights and support she has received from other caregivers she meets through the Stark Club and another support group for caregivers of people under sixty-five with Alzheimer's.

"I've been going to the under-sixty-five group for so long that I've seen a lot of new people," she says. "It helps me, seeing that I've made it to the point we are now. I didn't think I could do this a year ago. Two years ago, I saw other people who were further along and thought, 'I can't do that.' Two years later, I can do that. I'm here and I'm doing it."

Not that it's easy, Judy concedes. She has had to learn patience, she says. Sometimes she gets overwhelmed. Sometimes she cries. But she has also learned to reach out when she needs help and is blessed to have so many people who love her and Delbert, who are right nearby and anxious to help. "I sometimes feel like I have to do it all," she says. "But when I get to the point when I'm just about to break, I think about all the people who love and care for me and Delbert."

The loving family who surround Judy and Delbert are a model for the power of love to keep joy alive through hardship.

"We don't wish this difficult and heart-wrenching experience on anyone," Cathey says. "But for anyone who has to deal with Alzheimer's, our prayer would be that their family rallies around them as our family has to support Delbert. We have all learned so much from him, and he holds a special place in our hearts. We love him and are grateful to have him as such a special part of our family."

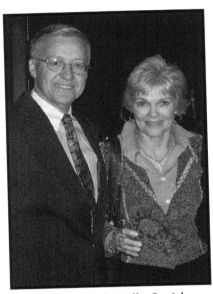

Wayne and Molly Smith

The qualities that made Wayne Smith the kind of man people loved and respected were not dimmed by Primary Progressive Aphasia.

Chapter 12
A Natural Leader

"A man is only as good as his word."
Wayne Smith

Wayne Smith exudes quiet power. A retired Navy admiral, Wayne stands for honesty and integrity. He was a founding member of the Stark Club who remained connected to the group even after he moved to Northern Virginia.

When Wayne walks into the room, I always feel like I should sit up a little straighter. Wayne is a gentle and good-natured person with a manner of authority and power, which is more striking because of his unassuming nature. Everyone who meets Wayne wants to make him proud.

Wayne was a founding member of the Stark Club, before I started working with the group. I used to see him and his attractive wife, Molly, at the center. They were always so bright, optimistic, and happy. I could feel the warmth of their personalities even in our casual acquaintance. After I started working with the Stark Club and got to know Wayne better, it was easy for me to understand why he achieved the rank of admiral. He doesn't demand attention, but people are drawn to him. He's quiet, but when he speaks he has something valuable to say. He's the kind of man who inspires you to do your best and the kind of man who, once he touches your life, stays in your heart forever. Wayne and Molly ultimately moved away and stopped attending Stark Club meetings, but none of us ever stopped thinking of him as an important member of the group.

———

Molly and Wayne were small-town Texas teenagers when they met, but Molly recognized the young man's potential immediately. "I knew he had all the qualities I would want in someone that I married," she says. "Wayne had good manners. He was respectful of other people, no matter who they were. And he put honesty above everything—for Wayne, a good person doesn't lie."

Wayne was easygoing and "middle of the road," in his younger days. "He enjoyed life," Molly says. He studied graphic arts and was an average student who wasn't interested enough in the field to try and excel. He graduated during the Vietnam War era and joined the Navy to avoid being drafted into the Army. After Naval Officer Candidate School, he immediately stepped into a work environment of older, more experienced Naval officers, most of whom had worked their way up through the ranks from enlisted personnel. But Wayne's quiet confidence and respect for others quickly made him a successful leader among older and more experienced officers. "He was wise for his years, and he always had great people skills," Molly says. "People have often said to me, 'I would go anywhere and do anything for your husband.'"

Wayne never resorted to yelling or using bad language to get his way or make a point and had little use for people who behaved childishly. And when he was displeased with something or someone, "You could tell by the look on his face," Molly says.

Wayne's personal code of conduct could even be a little difficult for friends and his son, Colby, to live up to. From the time Colby was old enough to understand, Wayne taught him to hold honesty above all else and often reminded Colby that "a man was only as good as his word."

Life was good for the Smiths, but in retrospect, Molly recalls hints of trouble in the 1990s that they dismissed. She remembers Wayne struggling to order at fast food restaurants. "He would get the order so screwed up that we would just burst out laughing," Molly remembers, adding that she would have to place the order. She also noticed that when Wayne talked on the telephone with other people, he had difficulty interjecting himself into the conversation.

Then he started having trouble with household chores. "The lawnmower broke and he couldn't fix it," Molly remembers. "He was like Tim the Toolman—nothing would go right for him. Simple things became a challenge. He would leave the garage door open or the back door open.

"Around Thanksgiving 1999, about a year and a half after his retirement, we were driving to East Texas and he said, 'I think I have Alzheimer's,'" Molly remembers. "I said, 'Oh no you don't.' But then he shared how that day at work, he'd had to give a speech and read something, but he couldn't do it. He couldn't read the words." Molly recalls thinking he may have something brain-related, but not Alzheimer's. Molly's father had died in January 1998 after a ten-year battle with Alzheimer's disease, and Wayne's symptoms seemed different.

From there, the couple did the familiar rounds. The doctors first tried antidepressants, theorizing that Wayne was depressed by the transition from the Navy to a civilian career after thirty-one years. "I thought, 'I'll go along with this diagnosis, but I don't buy it,'" Molly remembers. "Wayne would never get depressed, it wasn't in his character." Wayne was convinced the antidepressants would help. "He was so happy for awhile," Molly says. "I remember he told a close friend, 'I'm back and feeling great.'"

In December, Wayne's company went through a major reorganization and downsizing and offered him buyout package, which he took. Molly wasn't sure if Wayne was included because he was so junior, because his disease was affecting his work, or because of a combination of the two. Wayne began seeking employment with other companies and during this time, Molly stumbled upon an e-mail he had written. "It made no sense," she says. "The grammar was awful and when I approached him about it, he couldn't see anything wrong with it."

The next day Molly showed the e-mail to Wayne's psychiatrist, who immediately referred Wayne to a neurologist. The neurologist gave Wayne a preliminary examination and referred him for further testing.

Wayne underwent the testing with aplomb, remaining unrattled even when he couldn't accomplish a task. Doctors at Johns Hopkins University finally diagnosed Wayne with Primary Progressive Aphasia (PPA), at the age of fifty-four.

Wayne accepted the news stoically. "He showed disappointment but he never got down and out like I did," Molly says. Molly remembers taking the news hard, but people around her remember mostly the couple's grace under pressure.

At that time, we were in preliminary discussions about forming the Young Men's Group, later called the Stark Club. Wayne became one of the first members, along with Temple

Stark, Jerry Roach, and Alan Smith. At that time, Wayne was still in very early stages of PPA and able to contribute considerably to the group. He was also still driving then (he conscientiously took a driving test at Baylor to confirm that he was still OK to drive).

The men of the group bonded in that way men do—with easy, teasing banter. But the connection was deep and immediate. Sometimes I compare it to what I've heard about the camaraderie in the trenches of war. The men of the Stark Club understood the nuances of fighting the disease in a way that nobody else can, no matter how sympathetic.

Molly remembers that from the very first Stark Club meeting Wayne attended, he was impressed with the other members' intellect and humor. Wayne's sincere focus on others caused people to be naturally drawn to him. He was truly a born leader who didn't have to work at inspiring people; he emanated calm self-confidence and capability that signaled to all who met him that he was a man who could be trusted and respected.

Because Wayne's primary problem was with communication, Molly advised friends not to worry about Wayne responding to them, but to talk to him anyway. And she has commented that one particularly valuable aspect of the Stark Club was how members made Wayne feel as though nothing was ever out of the ordinary when he couldn't finish a sentence or say the right word. They didn't need patience to wait to for Wayne to articulate his thoughts because they had empathy. Wayne was the same way with others. He often approached other group members who had difficulty communicating and spent the time necessary for them to express their thoughts.

Wayne can be quiet in groups but garrulous one-on-one, even telling jokes. And he is always encouraging.

Some clichés just ring true: Wayne was an officer and a gentleman. The other men adored him. As for Wayne, "the Stark Club was his lifeline," Molly says. "It was the only thing in his life that would light him up, other than his son, daughter-in-law, and grandchildren."

———

As the disease progressed, Wayne continued adjusting stoically. Having heard that exercise was good for dementia and always conscious of his health, Wayne started running every morning after his diagnosis. The Smiths lived on a large property in a smallish Texas town and he loved to jog around the country. With his Navy training, Wayne's sense of direction was excellent. For a long time, he also was able to pursue his hobby of refinishing furniture and he helped around the house. He also worked uncrating food at the food bank in the town where they lived. In the midst of all the changes that were happening, Molly observed that Wayne and the other Stark Club members just "wanted to feel like they still fit in."

Wayne was very upset the Wednesday his neurologist suggested it was time for him to stop driving. Thursday evening, Molly says, he was still angry. But by Friday, when she came home from work, "he said, 'We're going to get rid of my truck and your car,'" Molly recalls. And that was that. He moved on. At his next appointment with his neurologist, Wayne apologized for being rude during his last visit, when she told him that he had her permission to stop driving. Once Wayne could no longer drive, Molly started taking a day off from work every other week to drive Wayne to Stark Club meetings.

———

In 2003, an excellent job opportunity presented itself to Molly and the couple decided to move to Washington, D.C. By this time, Wayne had been with the Stark Club for two years. I had only been working with the group for about six months and was enjoying the honor of getting to know Wayne. We were all sad to see him go.

We all made an effort to keep Wayne connected with our group. Shortly after the Smiths moved away, we sent him a photo of the group, which received a place of honor on his mantle, among family photos. Molly told me that Wayne would show it to their friends in D.C.

At various times, someone in the Stark Club would suggest we give Wayne a call. We would all crowd into my little office and use speaker phone to call his cell phone. One time we called him and he was outside walking in a park. He was so pleased to hear from us. I remember him saying once, "Is it everybody?" I had everyone say their names so he would know who was on the call.

On the calls, I would share bits of information I knew about him or others in the Stark Club. They'd laugh all together and enjoy just hearing each others voices. After we called the first time, Molly told me that when she got home from work that day, Wayne had a big grin on his face. He was able to get her to understand that the Stark Club called him. It apparently made his day.

Once, Molly and Wayne surprised the Stark Club with a note updating us on a trip they took to see their son and his family and a picture of Wayne playing with his grandson in a sandbox. I read the card to the group, and we talked about Wayne and passed the picture around. After a big groundbreaking ceremony and party for the Center for BrainHealth's new headcourters in Dallas, Jack Kalling emailed photos of the event to Wayne and Molly. In a way, the note he sent with the photos is like a mini-Stark Club meeting, touching on the emotional, personal, medical and newsy.

From Jack K:

Molly and Wayne,

It was a great day!

Enjoy the photos.

The black guy was father of brain-injured child.

He spoke well and touches our hearts.

My daughters and two grandkids are in these photos.

How you are?

My PPA is progressing.

TCU-Miller gave up speech therapy and prepared me for next phase. I bought and customize a small Picture Communicator from www.interactivetherapy.com. Bob and Marie Eshbaugh bought one also.

Sincerely,

Jack

By the time Wayne and Molly came back to visit friends and family in Texas in July 2006, Wayne's PPA and Frontotemporal dementia had progressed. Molly told me that he did little any more but sit in the house and watch news. He rarely spoke. He had to stop running after he got lost and ended up running along a six-lane highway in Alexandria, Virginia.

Wayne and Molly came up to the center to say hello to us. Wayne had a big smile on his face that grew enormous when he saw Stephanie, who worked with the Stark Club the first two years. When he saw her, tears came to his eyes. All of us who saw them were moved by the reunion. For us, it was confirmation that the work we were doing was touching people's hearts.

And we were excited and honored when the Smiths' living legacy, Colby, decided to do something practical to honor his father. He cycled two hundred miles from Austin to Dallas to raise awareness of dementia and money for our research, but most importantly "to bring a smile to my dad's face." Wayne was not at the finish line, but family, friends, Stark Club members, students, clinicians, and researchers at the Center for BrainHealth excitedly welcomed Colby and the other riders at the end of their heartfelt trek.

"For us, the Center for BrainHealth and the Stark Club made a huge difference in our lives," Molly says. "It brought us together with new friends sharing the same brain-related diseases, and enabled us to find humor in the challenges that Wayne's disease forced us to face each day. I will always remain grateful, appreciative, and thankful for the impact the Center for BrainHealth had on our lives."

Wayne became a part of the Stark Club at a turning point in his life—when he was still able to totally connect with the other group members and when he most needed comrades for the road ahead. Wayne had spent his life as friend, mentor, and leader, and he was able to bring those qualities to the Stark Club in ways that touched everyone he met. And Molly, who stays upbeat and emits a positive light ("You have to laugh or you go crazy," is her credo for coping), remains a joy to be around, even as her life gets tougher. Even in adversity, Wayne and Molly set an example for living that everyone who meets them aspires to.

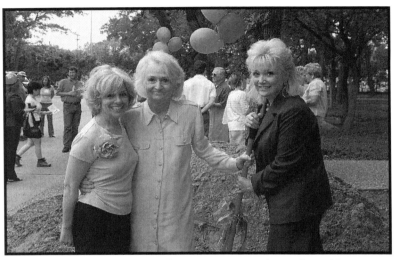

Sandi Chapman with Frances Goad Cecil and her daughter, Dianne Cash, at the groundbreaking of the Frances and Mildred Goad building.

Frances Goad Cecil lived her life with an open heart and irrepressible verve and Alzheimer's disease couldn't change that.

Chapter 13
A Generous Life

"Always be ready for a picnic."
Frances Goad Cecil

A modern woman and a genteel and spiritual Southern lady, Frances Goad Cecil was a working mother in an era when that was rare, and she kept a full calendar of volunteer work to satisfy her giving spirit. Frances possesses such a keen intellect that her Alzheimer's disease was advanced before anyone even realized something was wrong.

"There were eight of us…"

That's how Frances started all her many stories about growing up in a family of eight in small-town Oklahoma. It was an important time to her, and no matter how sophisticated she became after moving to Houston and then Dallas, she still retained solid, down-home roots.

Frances was a caretaker for her large family, and that is surely where she learned her empathetic ways and her astonishing self-possession. Frances is a raconteur—witty, charming, outgoing, warm, and smart. A tall, striking blonde and very much a lady in the time-honored, steel-magnolia, Southern style, Frances also was ahead of her time.

"Every single morning, Mother got up at 5:30, exercised thirty minutes—and this is when no one else did—read her Bible for an hour, then got dressed and went to work," remembers her daughter, Dianne Cash. Frances worked at Exxon all through Dianne's childhood, in an era when women more commonly stayed home. And she was always dressed like a lady in high heels, a skirt, pearls.

Widowed at forty-seven, Frances never remarried and worked hard to give Dianne a life full of opportunity and adventure. "We took a two- or three-week trip every summer," Dianne says. Frances always planned for a good time and nurtured a sense of excitement and adventure by saving money in a jar all year long for that year's upcoming trip. "I'd been in forty of the states before I was eight years old. I went to private school. I went to SMU (Southern Methodist University). Mother wanted me to have all that."

Frances also filled her life with extended family, friends, work, volunteerism, reading (and clipping items of interest to share with friends and family), and reaching out to others. "Mother was never idle, she never watched television," Dianne says. "She painted, gardened, and walked three to five miles every day until she was eighty-one. She was very much what I call a servant spirit. She always wanted to do for someone else. It was never about her. She was never self-centered, never egotistical, never demanding. She always had her pockets full of things to give people, but she never wanted anything in return. 'You can't out-give God,' she would say."

Frances had friends of all races, creeds, and social status and was a mentor to many. "She had no use for women who just played bridge," Dianne continues. "She said, 'You've got two legs, God gave you a brain, go do it.' She had no patience with people who want to whine and don't want to get out and do something."

The serene center of Frances' busy life was her spirituality. Her great grandfather was a circuit rider preacher and many other family members also were in the church. "That was the main thing Mother taught me early on," Dianne says. "When there was an issue, you'd just hit the floor on your knees."

Frances taught her loved ones a lot of things. "She did have opinions," Dianne says with an affectionate laugh, and she delights in reciting some of her mother's personal homilies—on health, for example. "She was always telling me, 'Dianne, eat more nuts.'" When Frances' many brothers and sisters moved to Houston one by one, she helped them get on their feet in many ways, including with oft-repeated advice to "get an apartment near the bus stop." And one of her favorite pieces of advice to women friends: "You need to wear a hat."

And while not advice, per se, Frances' response to anyone who asks how she was that day got a short response containing a complete philosophy: "Great," she'd say. "I saw the sun come up."

———

A mind as sharp and active as Frances' can often compensate with intelligence when the first symptoms of Alzheimer's start creeping up. Frances had lived so long doing all the right things—eating right, exercising, taking vitamins, keeping her mind and body active—Alzheimer's was practically unthinkable to all who knew her, despite the fact that two of her brothers had it.

But Frances knew.

"She was the one who said to me, 'Dianne, something is happening in my brain,'" Dianne recalls.

By the time Frances brought it up, Dianne was also wondering if something was wrong. "I started noticing," she says. "My grandmother had it and nobody would listen to me. She had to get into late stages before anybody ever got it. But I was on the lookout with Mother. I started noticing behavioral changes. She got more confrontational. She got lost sometimes."

As soon as Frances acknowledged that she was having problems, she and Dianne started consulting doctors. But Frances breezed through a couple of cognitive evaluations and the doctors dismissed her fears. "She was so funny and so sharp they always said, 'Oh, your mother is so great,'" Dianne recalls. "She'd talk to them about the latest sports—Mother read the paper voraciously."

And so for another two years, the family continued as if nothing was wrong.

Eventually Dianne noticed Frances driving erratically and took her car away. But what she noticed most was a change in her demure mother's behavior.

"She was starting to say and do things she would never have said before," Dianne recalls. "She would never tell off-color stories or be confrontational in the past." They weren't drastic changes. "Only someone who knew her as well as I would notice," Dianne says, but they were unmistakable to her. "I saw her every day, but I knew that she wasn't willing to go through further testing at the time."

Finally, though, Frances was distressed enough by changes and struggles she noticed in herself to agree to more testing. Frances and Dianne came to the Center for BrainHealth in 2001. Once again, specialists were amazed by Frances' sharp mind and wit. But they were then stunned to look at an MRI scan of her brain, which showed how advanced the disease actually was. "The hippocampus was pretty much gone," Dianne recalls. "They were shocked. They said this just doesn't happen."

———

Because Frances was in her eighties, we first tried her in a group of individuals of a similar age range, but we quickly realized that for Frances, age was just a number. We decided to invite Frances to the Stark Club and she immediately became a force to be reckoned with in the meetings. When Frances arrived, the energy in the room was palpable. Out of her purse would appear a box of chocolates to celebrate a birthday or a collection of jokes for the group. Frances always seemed to turn our meetings into little parties, and she felt it her job to keep spirits up and conversation lively. We never knew what she had planned for the group.

Her habit of pulling surprises out of her purse was not a new one, as I would later learn from Dianne. Frances lived by the credo that in life, one should "always be ready for a picnic." She celebrated life every day and always had a small gift or box of chocolates in her purse ready to brighten someone's day.

Frances' warm heart was evident in the Stark Club as well. She truly admired each member of the group and was always ready with a smile, hug, or encouraging word.

While having her mother remain as sharp as she did was wonderful for Dianne, it also required some creative thinking and thoughtful framing of the situation in order to keep her mother active and stimulated, while not underestimating the effects of the disease.

Frances continued living in her own home for two years after the diagnosis. The fact that she was a woman of regular habits helped her remain independent, since predictability and order are key to the comfort of people with Alzheimer's. She remained very active, still seeing friends, going to church, going to the symphony, and as always, she "turned out like a lady," Dianne says. "Mother had the best, given a crummy situation."

Dianne made a point of visiting Frances every day as the sun went down. "As the sun goes down, people with Alzheimer's get more forgetful, more confused. I always went to see her at about twilight because I wanted to see the worst part of the day, which would tell me where she really was in terms of the disease," Dianne explains. "I could pretty much tell when I walked into her house what kind of mood she was in by her face. I could sense if she was going to be really testy with me and argumentative."

Early on, Dianne sometimes found herself squabbling with Frances even though she knew that much of her mother's argumentativeness was the disease talking. "I would go home and say, 'Dianne, why did you say anything?'" Dianne recalls. "I went over every day. Many days I would get in the car and scream all the way home. Some days I'd cry on the way home."

Dianne knew intellectually that it was futile to argue with people with Alzheimer's, but occasionally disagreements would happen. Frances' sister, Marilyn, always kept their interactions light and fun. If Frances started arguing, Marilyn would lightheartedly say, "Oh, hush." Only once did Dianne take something Frances said to her personally.

"It hurt my feelings," she recalls. But otherwise, "Mother was always my best friend."

Dianne also learned to back off when Frances wanted more space, and to err on the side of giving her mother autonomy. Once, Frances scolded Dianne to "quit asking me if I have to go to the bathroom. I will tell you if I need to go to the bathroom."

———

Eventually, it became clear that she could no longer live alone, and Dianne looked for a care facility that would meet her high standards. "That was not something I was ever going to do, but I must admit that after I did it, life was a lot easier," Dianne says.

Dianne is fortunate to have the financial wherewithal to supply her mother with the best, and she took the time to make sure that everything was to her liking. "I'm very detail-oriented. If I were not, a lot of things would not have happened as well as I would have wanted them to," Dianne says. She found a facility just a half-mile from her home and got Frances a quiet corner room, which she decorated with photos and other personal belongings. "It's as familiar as I knew how to make it."

Dianne was unsatisfied with staff interactions she witnessed at the facility, so she decided to hire private caregivers for her mother, interviewing several and trying a few out before settling on four women. "I have people with her 24-7 so she's never alone," Dianne says. "I call them the 'Fab Four.' They're crazy about mother and she's crazy about them. They treat her like a queen. I culled through about twenty people to find them. Some were flippant, some didn't want to work, they just wanted to order pizza in, some wouldn't talk to mother, some would argue with her."

Dianne particularly likes the fact that the Fab Four always took the time to make sure Frances is turned out the way she would want to be, in coordinated outfits with jewelry, and her hair done.

Frances had many visitors at the care facility, including Dianne's children and grandchildren, and her old friend, Charlie, who visited daily. As Frances grew more cognitively impaired, Dianne made sure that she still lived a life of grace. When she realized Frances could no longer dine with higher functioning residents of the facility because it took her so long to eat (and they politely would sit with her until she was finished), Dianne asked for meals to be delivered to Frances' room rather than having her eat with people who were more profoundly impaired.

As time went on, the belligerent phase of Frances' disease passed and, after ten years of being uncharacteristically hard to get along with, she softened again, becoming "the sweet person she always was," Dianne said happily. "I saw that fighter for ten years. You do that long enough, you start thinking that's the person she always was. But then she was sweet again and I could love on her."

———

Dianne, a staunch supporter of the Center for BrainHealth and our mission, made a major donation towards our new facility to honor her mother and grandmother.

"As mother fades, the building will be there. I know that pleased her so much," Dianne said.

In October of 2006, the Center for BrainHealth moved into the beautiful Mildred and Frances Goad building.

Unfortunately, by this time Frances had suffered a series of strokes that greatly affected her health and cognitive functioning. As I was working on this chapter, Frances passed away.

Frances' funeral was a spirited celebration of a remarkable woman's life, with singing and stories and hundreds of people who came to give back the love that Frances had given to them.

I was unfortunately out of town the day of Frances' funeral, but in her honor that day, I wore a hat and ate nuts. The very least I could do to honor a woman who had touched me deeply was to follow her advice.

Frances lived her life with hope and faith to the very end.

"She did not complain or whine or say, 'Why did this happen to me?' Although she could have," Dianne said. "But she never did."

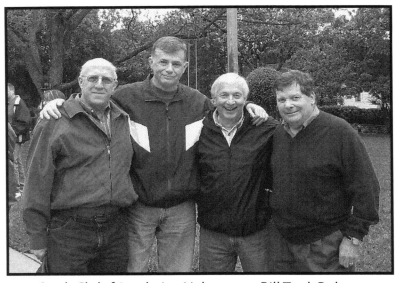

Stark Club friends Jay Haberman, Bill Tuel, Robert Eshbaugh, and Bill Crist

Stark Club members prove that life does not end with a diagnosis. They hope you will find hope and strength through their stories.

Chapter 14
Reframing Dementia

"Hope should be the last thing to ever die."
Dr. Sandra Chapman, UTD Center for BrainHealth

The Stark Club members chose to write this book to help others dealing with a diagnosis of Alzheimer's disease or other dementia. Following are a few lessons Stark Club members hope you gain from their stories.

Life continues despite the diagnosis. In an effort to be clear and direct, doctors often deliver the diagnosis of Alzheimer's in a manner that seems to preclude all hope. Know this: a diagnosis of Alzheimer's does not need to be a death sentence. Your life can continue to be rich, fulfilled, and happy after the diagnosis. Take advantage of the time you have to pursue the things you enjoy. Travel, spend time with friends, and continue to fill your days with wonderful memories.

Expect good days and bad days with Alzheimer's. We all have good days and bad days, including people with

Alzheimer's. The difference is, bad days are more obvious because the person has less ability to compensate. Take advantage of good days by doing something you enjoy, and pull back on bad days.

 Maintain social connections. Keep life as normal as possible by nurturing friendships and continuing favorite activities.

 Beware of "learned helplessness," when people quit doing things because nothing is expected of them. Keep individuals engaged by expecting their continued involvement.

Men with Alzheimer's still need male companionship. Most often women are found in the role of caregiver, especially professional caregivers. Men with Alzheimer's often have a life consisting of one female after another providing care. Friends stop coming around because they don't know how to handle it. It's up to the family to educate friends on how to stay involved.

Seek to maintain a sense of normalcy in life. "I think our efforts to maintain a sense of normalcy in life is what's kept Temple going as long as he's been going. We don't act like there's something wrong. We continue to live life," Anne Stark says.

Get a new perspective. The best lessons are caught, not taught. Find inspiration by surrounding yourself with people who move forward with hope.

Seek out and accept help early. Establish a network of friends and support before you need it so it is in place when you do.

Provide verbal guidance. When individuals are unable to do chores or activities on their own, provide verbal guidance or do projects together to prolong their involvement.

Don't borrow trouble from the future. This disease progresses slowly providing the opportunity to make adjustments in stages. Make decisions based on "what is" rather than living in a world of "what ifs." Focus on all the ways you can continue to appreciate each other today and have a fulfilling life.

Celebrate the person. Instead of focusing on what is impaired, focus on what the individual enjoys and still can do.

Find ways to promote communication without words. Some individuals with PPA are unable to verbalize information, but they can write it down. Jodi always carries a yellow pad with her to help her communicate. Encourage people with PPA to use communication aids such as drawing, using photographs to set the context, sharing brochures from events, or newspaper articles.

Support comprehension. Comprehension is intact in the early stage of PPA, but as PPA progresses, don't assume the person with the disease understands everything you say. Comprehension will be better for personal information or familiar topics. Use pictures or objects to help support the message you are trying to communicate. Keep the person involved by being a compassionate communicator.

Focus on the relationship. When communication breaks down, it's tempting to focus on the details of life and lose sight of quality of life both for the person with dementia and the family.

Become an advocate. Because a diagnosis of Alzheimer's disease is not expected in individuals under sixty, symptoms may go undiagnosed or misdiagnosed, requiring families to be persistent in understanding the signs and finding the cause for problems in memory and functioning. Carol says, "Looking back, I believe Bill showed signs of Alzheimer's at least five years before his diagnosis."

Educate yourself and others. Learn about the diagnosis, but don't focus on the negatives. Use this book to remind yourself of what you still can do. Sharing what you learn about living with Alzheimer's with others is a good way to open up communication about the disease.

Fight the stigma. When people hear the term "Alzheimer's disease," most people immediately think of the end stage. Hearing a message of hope from a person with the diagnosis is a powerful way to change perceptions.

Don't hide. It takes a lot of energy to keep a diagnosis a secret. You don't have to tell everyone, but being honest with family and friends will relieve a lot of pressure and help you focus on engaging in life.

Find ways to stay connected. Create a *Collection of Life Stories* to facilitate continued connection with family and friends. The book of stories is an incredible tool in facilitating continued socialization and celebrating the person.

Find your own solutions. "I feel very strongly you have to do what's right for the person and yourself," Shirley Kalling says. People and the dynamics in relationships differ; if a strategy doesn't work for you, evaluate why and create a solution that works for you.

Accept healthy denial. Denial is a challenge for the caregiver, but can help the person with dementia cope with the changes. Find ways to collaborate with the denial by bridging the gap between what they can do and what they think they can do.

Appreciate today. "Getting the diagnosis was so hard, but it seems we appreciate things like we never did before. Now we talk about the little details of the day and appreciate our time together more than ever. Alzheimer's has caused us to appreciate what we have and view every day as a gift," says Dawn.

Consider adopting a pet. Animals can be great companions and can add to quality of life with unconditional love and devotion that can help stave off moments of loneliness.

Don't sweat the small stuff. As much as possible, make an effort to defuse potentially stressful situations with a light-hearted response or by gently changing the focus of the conversation.

Remember, calm and quiet is good. High-energy situations and fast-moving conversations are stressful for individuals with dementia. Be aware of your environment and seek to minimize distractions.

Be liberal with encouragement. Sincere encouragement and words of appreciation mean a great deal to individuals with dementia and their care partners.

Offer help despite your fear. Many people feel awkward around individuals with Alzheimer's disease. When they consider reaching out as a friend or family member, their concern may be: "What do I do?" The answer is, do what you've always done and be willing to provide help if necessary.

Tap into long-term knowledge. It is amazing how many bits of information gathered over a lifetime are still accessible to a person with dementia. Take opportunities to talk about lifelong interests.

Focus on potential. Keep doing the things you do best and modify activities to promote continued involvement. Encourage friendships and participation in favorite activities.

Post Script

Since the writing of this book, we have lost many of the members of the Stark Club. But as I look back over the last nine years I realize how much these incredible people changed my perception of what it is to have and live with Alzheimer's disease. It is certainly not an easy path, but one that can be lived with dignity. I have the greatest respect for all the caregivers because this disease truly affects family relationships and friendships. The Stark Club members were proud to be a part of writing this book and for this experience, I will forever be grateful.

The Center for BrainHealth continues pursuing its mission of understanding, protecting and healing the brain.

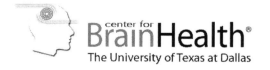

Made in the USA
Charleston, SC
29 January 2011